Anti-Inflammatory

Cookbook for Beginners

The complete guide to the anti-inflammatory diet, with many healthy recipes to reduce inflammation, balance hormones, and live a healthy life/30 Days meal plan.

Rachel Rodriguez

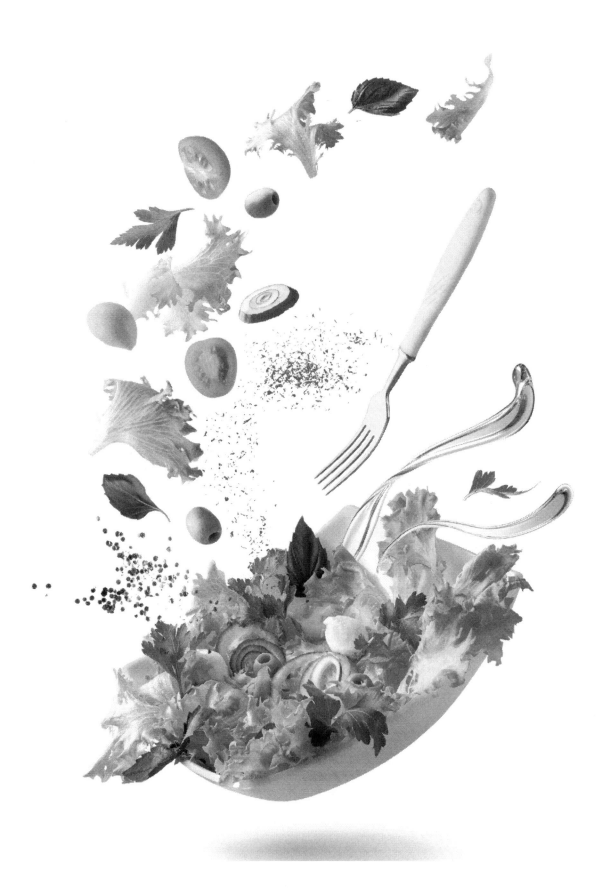

Table of Content

INTRODUCTION 10

CHAPTER 1: INFLAMMATION AND THE IMPORTANCE OF DIET 11

    1.1 WHAT IS INFLAMMATION? 11
    1.2 ACUTE INFLAMMATION VS. CHRONIC INFLAMMATION............................... 11
    1.3 CHRONIC INFLAMMATION AND CHRONIC DISEASES 12
    1.4 THE ROLE OF DIET IN INFLAMMATION 12
    1.5 THE PATH TO AN ANTI-INFLAMMATORY DIET 12

CHAPTER 2: BASIC PRINCIPLES OF THE ANTI-INFLAMMATORY DIET 13

    2.1 FOODS TO AVOID OR REDUCE..13
    2.2 FOODS TO INCLUDE 13
    2.3 IMPORTANCE OF HYDRATION 14
    2.4 BALANCE AND MODERATION 14

CHAPTER 3: FOODS AND NUTRIENTS WITH ANTI-INFLAMMATORY POWER...15

    3.1 FOODS RICH IN ANTIOXIDANTS 15
    3.2 OMEGA-3 FATTY ACIDS 16
    3.3 SPICES WITH ANTI-INFLAMMATORY POWER.......................................16
    3.5 THE CHALLENGE OF MEAL PREPARATION 16

CHAPTER 4: LIFESTYLE AND TIPS FOR OPTIMIZING THE ANTI-INFLAMMATORY DIET 17

    4.1 REGULAR PHYSICAL ACTIVITY 17
    4.2 QUALITY SLEEP 17
    4.3 STRESS MANAGEMENT 18
    4.4 MONITORING PROGRESS AND ADJUSTMENTS 18

CHAPTER 5: EXERCISE AND THE ANTI-INFLAMMATORY DIET: A WINNING COMBINATION 19

    5.1 THE EFFECTS OF EXERCISE ON INFLAMMATION...................................19
    5.2 CARDIOVASCULAR EXERCISE 20
    5.3 RESISTANCE EXERCISES 20
    5.4 YOGA AND STRETCHING... 20
    5.5 SAFETY CONSIDERATIONS 20
    5.6 JOINING FORCES: DIET AND EXERCISE... 20
    5.7 A PERSONALIZED APPROACH 20
    5.8 FREE-BODY EXERCISES THAT YOU CAN DO IN THE COMFORT OF YOUR OWN HOME WITHOUT THE NEED FOR EQUIPMENT. 21
        1. JUMPING JACKS (STAR JUMPING). 21
        2. PUSH-UPS (PUSH-UPS) 21
        3. SQUATS (SQUAT). 21
        4. LUNGES (LUNGES) 21
        5. PLANK (ISOMETRIC BRIDGE) 22

6. GLUTE BRIDGES (GLUTE BRIDGE). 22
7. SUPERMAN (SUPERMAN) 22
8. MOUNTAIN CLIMBERS. 22
9. TRICEP DIPS (PUSH-UPS FOR TRICEPS). 22
10. BIRD-DOG (HUNTING DOG) 23
11. SIDE PLANK (SIDE PLANK). 23
12. BICYCLE CRUNCHES (BICYCLE CRUNCHES). 23
13. JUMP SQUATS (JUMP SQUATS). 23
14. TRICEP PUSH-UPS (PUSH-UPS FOR TRICEPS). 23
15. BEAR CRAWL (BEAR WALK). 24
5.9 WEEKLY WORKOUT ROUTINES USING FREE-BODY EXERCISES...............24
***ROUTINE 1 - BEGINNER LEVEL**.* 24
***ROUTINE 2 - INTERMEDIATE LEVEL**.* 24
***ROUTINE 3 - ADVANCED LEVEL**.* 25
***ROUTINE 4 - FULL-BODY CIRCUIT**.* 25
***ROUTINE 5 - CORE FOCUS**.* 25
***ROUTINE 6 - HIGH-INTENSITY INTERVAL TRAINING (HIIT)**.* 26
***ROUTINE 7 - TOTAL BODY STRENGTH**.* 26
***ROUTINE 8 - ENDURANCE CHALLENGE**.* 26

CHAPTER 6: BREAKFAST RECIPES **28**
MUSHROOM QUINOA 29
BANANA CHIPS 29
COCONUT CREAM PANCAKES 29
MAYO SALAD 30
VEGETABLES QUINOA 30
BREAD WITH ALKALINE VEGETABLE CREAM 30
ZUCCHINI MUFFIN 30
CARROT JUICE 31
POTATO SALAD 31
BANANA PORRIDGE 31
BREAKFAST SALAD 31
BUTTERNUT SQUASH 32
ALKALINE MINESTRONE 32
LEMON SMOOTHIE 32
CABBAGE SALAD 33
RED THAI VEGETABLE CURRY 33
ZUCCHINI HOME FRIES 33
GREEN SMOOTHIE 34
HEMP SEED PORRIDGE 34

CHAPTER 7: LUNCH RECIPES **35**
ROASTED TOFU WITH COCONUT MILK 36
SWEET AND SOUR POTATOES WITH MEAT 36
STUFFED PEPPERS 36
BAKED FISH 37
ONION OMELETTE 37
CHICKPEAS AND VEGETABLES 37
BOILED CHICKEN 37

VEAL WITH MANGO SAUCE 38
BAKED TOMATOES 38
VEGETABLE HASH 38
CHAMPIGNON OMELETTE 39
CHICKEN WITH SWEET POTATOES 39
MIX GRILLED VEGETABLES 39
VEGETABLES AND LENTILS 40
ARTICHOKES AND QUINOA 40
STUFFED EGGPLANT 40
BAKED ONIONS AND POTATOES 41
SPICY MEAT 41
MIX FERMENTED VEGETABLES 41
ASPARAGUS OMELETTE 42
ROASTED EGGPLANT 42

CHAPTER 8: DINNER RECIPES 43

CILANTRO LIME QUINOA 44
SPINACH QUINOA 44
PINEAPPLE AND CARROT SALAD 44
PEPPERS PIZZA 45
HEALTHY BROCCOLI AND ASPARAGUS 45
BAKED PUMPKIN 45
PUMPKIN RISOTTO 45
MIXED LEGUMES SOUP 46
ZUCCHINI RISOTTO 46
PINEAPPLE AND COCONUT 47
CHICKEN MUFFIN 47
RAW RAINBOW VEGETABLES 47
FRESH FRUIT AND VANILLA 47
VEGETABLES WITH GREEN TOPPINGS 48
CHAMPIGNON RISOTTO 48
ROASTED ZUCCHINI 49
SWEET PEPPER CREAM 49
BANANA SMOOTHIE 49
BANANA AND COCONUT JUICE 49
TOMATO CREAM WITH QUINOA 50
GREEN SWEET CREAMY ZUCCHINI 50

CHAPTER 9: MAIN RECIPES 51

MASHED CAULIFLOWER 52
MEAT HASH 52
BEANS 52
QUINOA AND OATMEAL 52
SCRAMBLED TOFU E TOMATO 53
CHEESES AND QUINOA 53
SQUASH HASH 53
SWEET SQUID 53
ROASTED PEPPER CREAM 54
HOMEMADE MAYO 54

Octopus with green Sauce 54

Grilled Tofu 55

Fish Salad 55

Simple Carpaccio 55

CHAPTER 10: SIDES RECIPES 56

Grilled Vegetables 57

Coconut and mango 57

Simple Basil Quinoa 57

Vegetable Toast 57

Homemade Bread 58

Green anti-inflammatory roasted salad 58

Fresh Spelled Avocado Salad 58

Vegan spring roll 59

Vegetables Spring 59

Boiled Potato 59

Roasted Onion 60

Spinach with Garlic 60

Coconut and Avocado 60

Healthy Anti-inflammatory Salad 60

Sweet Beetroot 61

CHAPTER 11: SALAD RECIPES 62

Green Simple Salad 63

Tofu vegan Salad 63

Seitan Salad 63

Potatoes Salad 63

Radicchio Salad 64

Tomatoes Salad 64

Champignon Salad 64

Pumpkin Salad 65

Zucchini Salad 65

Boiled Endive Salad 65

Organic Meat Salad 65

Green Bean Salad 66

Yellow Salad 66

Legumes Mix Salad 66

CHAPTER 12: POULTRY RECIPES 67

Breaded Chicken 68

Chicken with green Sauce 68

Grilled Chicken 68

Spicy Chicken 68

Stuffed Chicken 69

Chicken with Pink Sauce 69

Cheese Chicken 69

Italian Chicken 70

Chicken Soup 70

Green Chicken 70

Chicken BBQ 71
Almond Chicken 71

CHAPTER 13: SEAFOOD RECIPES 72

Baked Sea Bass 73
Raw Tuna 73
Breaded Cod 73
Boiled Sea Bass 73
Smoked Salmon 74
Alkaline Sea Bass 74
Sea Salad 74
Pasta with Seafood 75
Boiled Octopus 75
Baked Squid 75
Rocket Fish 76
Roasted Salmon 76

CHAPTER 14: MEAT RECIPES 77

Simple Veal 78
Sweet and sour rabbit 78
Pork Stew 78
Roasted Veal 78
Baked Rabbit 79
Veal with alkaline Seasonings 79
Baked Pork 79
Boiled Veal 79
Pork with Green Sauce 80
Baked Turkey 80
Meat with peppers 80
Goat with eggplant 81

CHAPTER 15: SNACKS RECIPES 82

Detox Dried Fruit with Chestnut Honey 83
Chia Breadstick and cracker 83
Orange and Pumpkin Salad 83
Strawberry Salad 83
Biscuits bars 84
Chickpea Humus 84
Pear and Apple Extract 84
Fermented Zucchini 84
Purifying Juice 85
Avocado Salad 85

CHAPTER 16: SOUP RECIPES 86

Garlic soup 87
Onion Soup 87
Pepper Soup 87
Green Soup 88
cheeses Soup 88

BOILED VEGETABLES SOUP 88

SPINACH SOUP 88

MEAT SOUP 89

TURNIP SOUP 89

CHAPTER 17: VEGETABLES RECIPES 90

ANTI-INFLAMMATORY VEGETABLES 91

AVOCADO PIZZA 91

ANTI-INFLAMMATORY BROTH 91

CARROTS CREAM 91

AVOCADO AND EGGS SALAD 92

VEGETABLE CAKE 92

VEGETABLES PIZZA 92

VEGGIE DIPS 93

TOMATOES AND ZUCCHINI 93

CHAPTER 18: DESSERT RECIPES 94

CHOCOLATE COOKIES 95

COCONUT CREAM BARS 95

ALMOND CAKE 95

KIWI WITH DRIED FRUIT 95

HOMEMADE PROTEIN BARS 96

BANANA AND NUTS MUFFIN 96

STRAWBERRY JAM 96

SIMPLE ANTI-INFLAMMATORY BISCUIT 96

CEREAL WITH YOGURT 97

COCONUT CHIPS 97

APPLE CAKE 97

COCONUT AND ALMOND BISCUITS 97

APPLE MUFFIN 98

APPLE ALKALINE CREAM 98

YOGURT AND DRIED FRUIT 98

FANCY SPELT BREAD 99

LEMON ICE CREAM 99

ALMOND PARFAIT 99

NUT CREAM 99

AVOCADO CHIPS 100

CONVERSION CHART 101

30 DAY MEAL PLAN 102

CONCLUSION: 104

INTRODUCTION

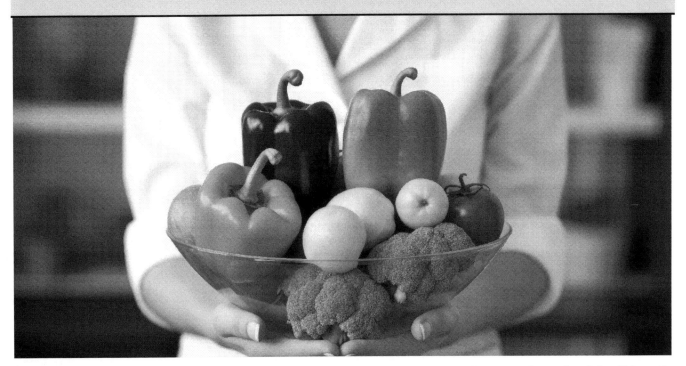

Welcome! I am Rachel Rodriguez, a nutritionist and passionate advocate for a healthy lifestyle through proper nutrition. I am excited to guide you on this journey to an anti-inflammatory diet, a nutritional approach that can significantly benefit your overall health and well-being.

As a health professional, I have seen countless times the positive impact an inflammation-targeted diet can have on people's lives. Chronic inflammation is often the underlying common denominator of many chronic diseases, and working to reduce it can make a big difference in preventing or managing these conditions.

In our track, we will explore the basics of inflammation, the critical role nutrition plays in controlling it, and how we can make intelligent choices to support our bodies in the healing process. Our daily diet should be seen not just as a means to appease hunger but as a powerful resource to promote health and vitality.

Through the following chapters, we will closely examine foods and nutrients with anti-inflammatory properties, learn to recognize those that may contribute to excessive inflammation, and discover strategies for adopting a healthy lifestyle to support an anti-inflammatory diet.

Remember that each individual is unique, with different needs and requirements, and this guide will only provide a base from which to start. You should consult with me or a health professional for a personalized assessment to help you develop an eating plan tailored to your specific needs.

Are we ready to embark on this journey together? Let's discover how to make food choices that will move us closer to a healthier life with less inflammation and more energy to face each day with vitality. Let's take care of ourselves through food, the first step to better health!

CHAPTER 1: INFLAMMATION AND THE IMPORTANCE OF DIET

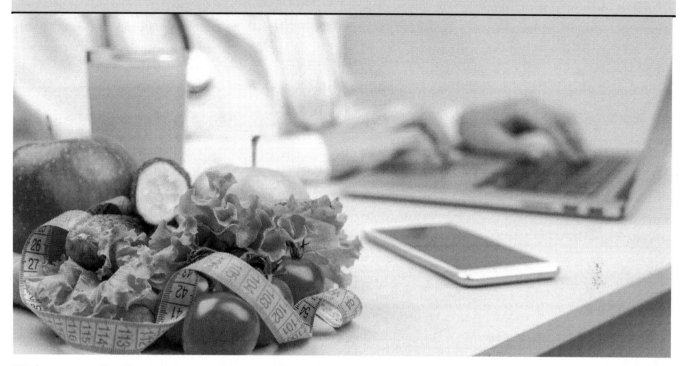

Welcome to the first chapter of our guide to the anti-inflammatory diet. We begin this journey by exploring inflammation and its critical role in our bodies, as well as the crucial impact that an appropriate diet can have on its management.

1.1 WHAT IS INFLAMMATION?

Inflammation is a natural response of our immune system to situations of stress, injury, or infection. When the body detects a potential threat, the immune system sends cells and chemicals to protect and repair damaged tissue. This process is known as acute inflammation and is essential for healing and recovery.

1.2 ACUTE INFLAMMATION VS. CHRONIC INFLAMMATION

Acute inflammation is usually short-term and resolves once the emergency has passed. However, chronic inflammation can become chronic due to modern lifestyles, including an unhealthy diet, chronic stress, lack of physical activity, and harmful habits. This constant and persistent inflammation can become detrimental to the body and is associated with many chronic diseases, such as type 2 diabetes, heart disease, arthritis, and many others.

1.3 CHRONIC INFLAMMATION AND CHRONIC DISEASES

Chronic inflammation can be a trigger or contributor to the development of several chronic diseases. For example, excess adipose tissue produces inflammatory substances, increasing overall inflammation in the body and promoting the development of metabolic problems, such as insulin resistance and type 2 diabetes. In addition, chronic inflammation can damage artery walls, leading to atherosclerosis and increasing the risk of cardiovascular disease.

1.4 THE ROLE OF DIET IN INFLAMMATION

Diet plays a crucial role in the management of chronic inflammation. Some foods can increase inflammation, while others can help reduce it. Choosing foods rich in antioxidants, vitamins, and minerals and the proper proportion of healthy fats, proteins, and complex carbohydrates can help balance inflammation and promote better health.

1.5 THE PATH TO AN ANTI-INFLAMMATORY DIET

In the remainder of our guide, we will explore the basic principles of an anti-inflammatory diet. We will learn which foods to include in our daily diet and which to avoid to reduce chronic inflammation and improve overall well-being. We will also explore the importance of hydration, omega-3 fatty acids, and spices with anti-inflammatory power.

Are you ready to discover how food can become your ally in the fight against chronic inflammation? Let's move on to the next chapter, where we will explore the basics of the anti-inflammatory diet and how to start making informed food choices for better health and well-being.

CHAPTER 2: BASIC PRINCIPLES OF THE ANTI-INFLAMMATORY DIET

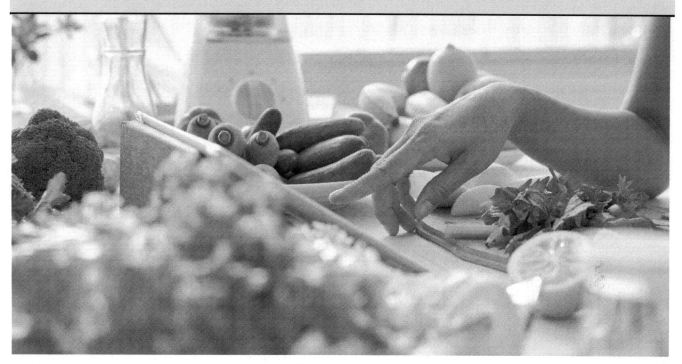

Welcome to the second chapter of our guide to the anti-inflammatory diet. This chapter will delve into the essential principles for creating a diet that promotes reducing chronic inflammation in our bodies. We will determine which foods to include and which to avoid to support our immune system and promote optimal health.

2.1 FOODS TO AVOID OR REDUCE

To begin the journey toward an anti-inflammatory diet, limiting or eliminating certain foods that may contribute to inflammation in our bodies is crucial. Some of these foods include:
- Processed foods that are high in saturated and trans fats.
- Refined sugars and simple carbohydrates, such as sweets, sugary drinks, and baked goods.
- Trans fats, often found in fried foods and industrial foods.
- Foods with a high glycemic index can raise blood sugar levels and promote inflammation.

2.2 FOODS TO INCLUDE

On the other hand, many foods can help reduce inflammation and promote overall health. Our diet should include:
- Fruits and vegetables are rich in antioxidants, vitamins, and minerals that help fight inflammation. Berries, citrus fruits, spinach, broccoli, and avocados are some antioxidant-rich foods.

- Lean sources of protein: lean meats, fish, poultry, legumes, and tofu are good sources of protein that help build and repair tissue without contributing to inflammation.
- Healthy fats: omega-3 fatty acids found in fatty fish such as salmon and sardines, flaxseed, and fish oil are known for their anti-inflammatory properties. Vegetable oils such as extra virgin olive oil also contain healthy fats that promote heart health and reduce inflammation.
- Whole grains: brown rice, quinoa, oats, and other whole grains are rich in fiber and health-beneficial nutrients and can help reduce inflammation.

2.3 IMPORTANCE OF HYDRATION

Keeping properly hydrated is essential for the optimal functioning of our bodies. Water helps eliminate toxins and promotes the circulation of nutrients. Drink enough water throughout the day and consider including green tea or herbal teas, which can provide additional anti-inflammatory benefits.

2.4 BALANCE AND MODERATION

An anti-inflammatory diet is not based on a single food category but on overall balance. Choose foods from different food categories and remember to moderate portions. Maintaining a balance of protein, carbohydrates, and fat will help you achieve a sustainable, healthy diet over time.

Continue with your enthusiasm and get ready to explore specific foods and nutrients with anti-inflammatory powers in the next chapter. Let food become your medicine as you move toward reduced inflammation and a better quality of life!

CHAPTER 3: FOODS AND NUTRIENTS WITH ANTI-INFLAMMATORY POWER

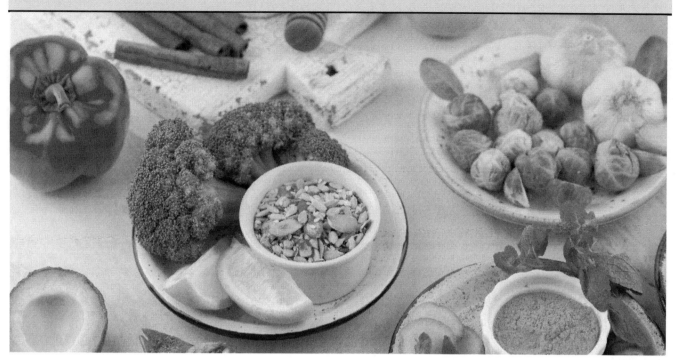

Welcome to the third chapter of our guide to the anti-inflammatory diet. In this chapter, we will explore in detail the foods and nutrients shown to possess anti-inflammatory properties, helping us reduce inflammation in our bodies and promote long-term health.

3.1 FOODS RICH IN ANTIOXIDANTS

Antioxidants are potent allies in the fight against inflammation. They neutralize free radicals, unstable molecules that can damage cells in our bodies, contributing to inflammation and premature aging. Some foods rich in antioxidants include:
- Berries such as blueberries, strawberries, raspberries and cranberries.
- Citrus fruits such as oranges, lemons, and grapefruits.
- Dark green leafy vegetables such as spinach and kale.
- Dried fruits such as walnuts and almonds.
- Green tea and matcha tea.

3.2 OMEGA-3 FATTY ACIDS

Omega-3 fatty acids are known for their anti-inflammatory properties and role in promoting heart and brain health. They can help balance inflammation in our bodies by reducing the production of inflammatory substances. Some foods rich in omega-3 include:
- Fatty fish such as salmon, mackerel, sardines, and herring.
- Flaxseeds and flaxseed oil.
- Nuts and seeds such as walnuts, chia, and hemp seeds.

3.3 SPICES WITH ANTI-INFLAMMATORY POWER

Spices are a delicious way to flavor our dishes while gaining anti-inflammatory benefits. Some of the spices with anti-inflammatory properties include:
- Turmeric: contains curcumin, a powerful compound with anti-inflammatory properties.
- Ginger: has antioxidant and anti-inflammatory properties.
- Cinnamon: can help reduce inflammation and stabilize blood sugar levels.

3.4 Importance of a varied and colorful diet
To get the maximum benefit from the anti-inflammatory diet, consuming a wide range of nutritious and colorful foods is essential. Each food group offers different nutrients and antioxidants, and combining various foods ensures we get all possible benefits.

3.5 THE CHALLENGE OF MEAL PREPARATION

Preparing healthy and nutritious meals may seem like a challenge, but it can be made easier with planning and organization. Take time to plan your weekly meals, buy fresh ingredients, and batch cook whenever possible. Also, explore anti-inflammatory recipes to make the meal preparation process more inspiring and tasty.

Get ready for the next chapter, in which we will explore the link between a healthy lifestyle and the management of chronic inflammation. You will discover the importance of regular physical activity, quality sleep, and stress management to support an anti-inflammatory diet and optimal health. Let's continue our journey to wellness together!

CHAPTER 4: LIFESTYLE AND TIPS FOR OPTIMIZING THE ANTI-INFLAMMATORY DIET

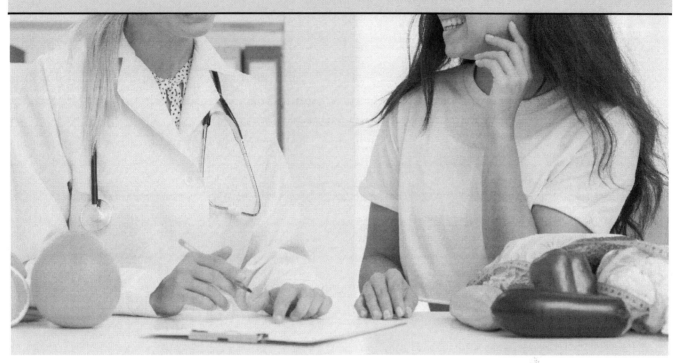

Welcome to the fourth chapter of our guide to the anti-inflammatory diet. In this chapter, we will explore the importance of lifestyle in supporting an anti-inflammatory diet and how certain daily habits can affect chronic inflammation in our bodies.

4.1 REGULAR PHYSICAL ACTIVITY

Regular exercise is a critical element of overall health and well-being, as well as chronic inflammation management. Physical activity can reduce inflammation levels in the body and improve insulin sensitivity, thus helping to control blood sugar levels. Combining cardiovascular exercises, such as walking, swimming, or cycling, with resistance exercises, such as weightlifting, can be particularly effective in combating inflammation.

4.2 QUALITY SLEEP

Quality sleep is essential for overall health and for controlling inflammation. During sleep, the body repairs and regenerates; a lack of sleep can increase inflammation levels. We get 7 to 9 hours of sleep each night by creating a relaxing bedtime routine, avoiding electronic devices before bedtime, and maintaining a comfortable temperature in the bedroom.

4.3 STRESS MANAGEMENT

Chronic stress is another factor that can contribute to inflammation in the body. Stress management is critical to our overall well-being and keeping inflammation under control. Find activities that help you relax and reduce stress, such as meditation, yoga, walking outdoors, or a hobby you enjoy. Making time for yourself and practicing stress management techniques can make a big difference in maintaining balance.

4.4 MONITORING PROGRESS AND ADJUSTMENTS

Every individual is different, and responses to diet and lifestyle changes may vary. Monitoring progress is essential to understand how your anti-inflammatory diet is working. Keep a food diary to record what you eat and how you feel after meals. Pay attention to symptoms of chronic inflammation, such as bloating, joint pain, or fatigue, and notice any improvements as you change your diet.

CHAPTER 5: EXERCISE AND THE ANTI-INFLAMMATORY DIET: A WINNING COMBINATION

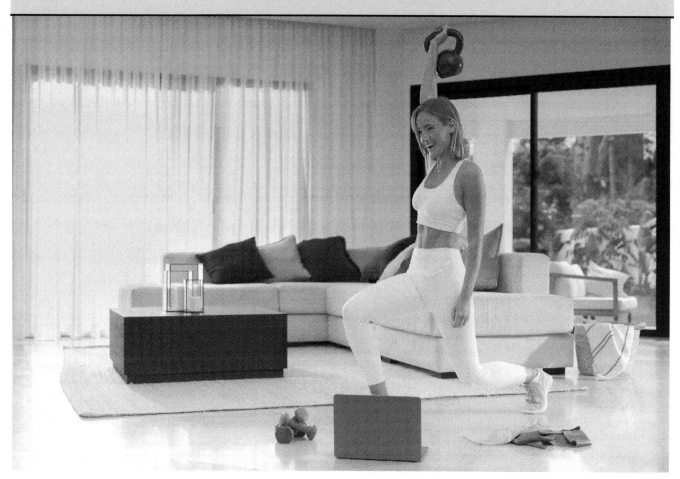

Welcome to the fifth chapter of our guide to the anti-inflammatory diet. In this chapter, we will explore the critical role of exercise when combined with an anti-inflammatory diet. We will discover how these two components can work synergistically to help reduce chronic inflammation in our bodies and promote optimal health.

5.1 THE EFFECTS OF EXERCISE ON INFLAMMATION

Regular exercise is a powerful tool for controlling inflammation in our bodies. During physical activity, physiological responses occur that help reduce inflammation. Moderate and constant exercise stimulates the release of anti-inflammatory molecules, helping to balance our body's inflammatory response.

5.2 CARDIOVASCULAR EXERCISE

Cardiovascular exercises like walking, running, swimming, or cycling are particularly effective in fighting inflammation. During cardiovascular activity, the heart pumps blood faster, increasing blood flow and tissue oxygenation. This process reduces oxidative stress and helps mitigate systemic inflammation.

5.3 RESISTANCE EXERCISES

Resistance exercises, such as weight lifting or free weights, can help reduce inflammation through several pathways. These exercises stimulate muscle growth and the release of anti-inflammatory substances, allowing counter-inflammation at the cellular level.

5.4 YOGA AND STRETCHING

Yoga and stretching practices can have a significant impact on inflammation management. These activities promote relaxation and can help reduce the stress hormone cortisol, which can increase inflammation when produced in excess. In addition, peace and the release of muscle tension improve blood circulation, promoting the transport of nutrients and the elimination of toxins from the body.

5.5 SAFETY CONSIDERATIONS

Before embarking on any exercise program, it is essential to consider your health and your current level of physical activity. If you have safety concerns or pre-existing medical conditions, I recommend that you consult a qualified health professional or personal trainer before beginning a new exercise regimen. A gradual, progressive approach is often the key to getting the benefits of exercise without risking injury or overload.

5.6 JOINING FORCES: DIET AND EXERCISE

Combining an anti-inflammatory diet with a regular exercise program can experience even more significant results. Diet provides our bodies with the tools to fight inflammation, while exercise helps optimize the anti-inflammatory response.

5.7 A PERSONALIZED APPROACH

Remember that each individual is unique, and the type of exercise best suited for you may vary. Find a physical activity that you enjoy, and that fits your lifestyle. The goal is to make exercise part of your daily routine and enjoy the process so you can maintain it over the long term.

In conclusion, exercise is essential for managing inflammation and achieving optimal health. Combined with an anti-inflammatory diet, it can help significantly improve your overall well-being. Keep committed to exploring the marriage of healthy eating and physical activity, and you will see your body and mind thank you with renewed vitality and energy.

5.8 FREE-BODY EXERCISES THAT YOU CAN DO IN THE COMFORT OF YOUR OWN HOME WITHOUT THE NEED FOR EQUIPMENT.

Always warm up properly before starting any workout, and consult a health professional if you have concerns about your physical fitness.

1. JUMPING JACKS (STAR JUMPING).

- Starting Position: Standing with legs together and arms along your sides.
- Movement: Jump by opening your legs to the side while raising your arms above your head. Return to starting position by jumping again. Repeat the movement smoothly and continuously.
- Benefits: This exercise helps warm the body by engaging the heart and muscles. It is a great cardiovascular exercise to start your exercise session.

2. PUSH-UPS (PUSH-UPS)

- Starting Position: Stand face down with your hands on the floor just outside shoulder width and your legs extended behind you.
- Movement: Lower your body by bending your elbows and lowering yourself toward the floor. Keep your body in a straight line without turning your back. Push the body upward, returning to the starting position.
- Benefits: Push-ups are an excellent exercise for the chest, shoulders, triceps, and abs, strengthening the upper body.

3. SQUATS (SQUAT).

- Starting Position: Stand with feet shoulder-width apart, toes pointing slightly outward.
- Movement: Bend your knees and lower your pelvis downward as if you were sitting on an invisible chair. Keep your weight on your heels, and make sure your knees do not go past the tips of your toes. Return to a standing position by pushing through the heels.
- Benefit: Squats engage the leg, gluteal and abdominal muscles, helping to strengthen the legs and improve balance.

4. LUNGES (LUNGES)

- Starting position: Standing with feet shoulder-width apart.
- Movement: Step forward with one leg, lowering the knee of the back leg toward the floor, without letting the knee touch the ground. Ensure your front knee is aligned with your ankle and your weight is distributed between your heel and toe. Return to the starting position and repeat with

the other leg.
- Benefit: Lunges work the legs, glutes, and hip muscles, helping to improve strength and stability.

5. PLANK (ISOMETRIC BRIDGE)

- Starting Position: Stand face down with your elbows resting on the floor below your shoulders and your toes extended behind you.
- Movement: Lift your body so that it is in a straight line from head to toe, keeping your core contracted and your glutes tight. Hold this position for as long as desired, keeping your back flat and neck in a neutral position.
- Benefits: The plank is an excellent core-stabilizing exercise, engaging the abdominals, lower back, and shoulder muscles.

6. GLUTE BRIDGES (GLUTE BRIDGE).

- Starting position: Lying on your back with knees bent and feet resting on the floor, close to the buttocks. Arms are extended along the sides.
- Movement: Lift your pelvis upward, pushing your heels to the floor and contracting your glutes. Keep your upper body and shoulders on the floor, creating a straight line between your knees, hips, and shoulders. Pause at the top and then return to the starting position.
- Benefit: This exercise is excellent for strengthening the glutes and lower back, improving core stability.

7. SUPERMAN (SUPERMAN)

- Starting Position: Lie on your stomach with your arms stretched out in front of you and your legs long.
- Movement: Simultaneously lift your arms, chest, and legs off the floor, creating a "U" shape with your body. Hold the position for a few seconds and then return to the starting position.
- Benefits: This exercise strengthens the lower back, improving posture and core stability.

8. MOUNTAIN CLIMBERS.

- Starting Position: Get into a plank position, with your palms resting on the ground below your shoulders and your toes stretched out behind you.
- Movement: Bring your right knee toward your chest, then return to the plank position. Repeat the movement with your left leg. Alternate legs quickly as if you were running in a horizontal position.
- Benefits: This exercise is a great cardiovascular workout, engaging the muscles of the heart, legs, and arms.

9. TRICEP DIPS (PUSH-UPS FOR TRICEPS).

- Starting position: Sit in a chair or on a stable bench with hands resting on the edge, fingers pointing down. Your legs are bent with your feet on the floor.
- Movement: Lift your body off the chair by bending your elbows downward, then return to the

starting position. Keep your shoulders close to your body, and your elbows pointed backward during the movement.
- Benefit: This exercise strengthens the triceps, arms, and shoulders.

10. BIRD-DOG (HUNTING DOG)

- Starting Position: Stand on all fours, with your hands under your shoulders and knees under your hips.
- Movement: Extend your right arm forward and left leg backward, keeping your back straight. Hold the position for a few seconds, then return to the starting position and repeat with the other arm and leg.
- Benefit: This exercise helps improve core stability and coordination while engaging the back and leg muscles.

11. SIDE PLANK (SIDE PLANK).

- Starting Position: Get into a left-side plank position, with your left elbow resting below your shoulder and your legs stretched out on each other.
- Movement: Lift your pelvis off the floor, forming a straight line from head to toe. Hold this position for a few seconds and then return to the starting position. Repeat on the right side.
- Benefits: The side plank strengthens the obliques, improving core stability and lateral strength.

12. BICYCLE CRUNCHES (BICYCLE CRUNCHES).

- Starting position: Lie on your back with hands behind your head and knees bent. Bring your legs above the floor so your thighs are perpendicular.
- Movement: Bring your right knee toward your chest while at the same time rotating your torso by bringing your left elbow toward your right knee. Then, extend the right leg backward and bring the left knee toward the chest while rotating the torso bringing the right elbow toward the left knee. Continue to repeat the movement smoothly and energetically.
- Benefit: This exercise engages the oblique abdominals, helping to tone the abs and improve core stability.

13. JUMP SQUATS (JUMP SQUATS).

- Starting Position: Standing with feet shoulder-width apart.
- Movement: Perform a squat by bending your knees and lowering yourself toward the floor. Upon returning to standing, perform a jump squat by extending your arms above your head. Land softly and bend your knees again to start the next squat.
- Benefits: Jump squats increase heart rate, engaging the leg muscles and helping to improve cardiovascular endurance.

14. TRICEP PUSH-UPS (PUSH-UPS FOR TRICEPS).

- Starting position: Get into a plank position with your hands close together, directly under your shoulders. Forearms are parallel to each other.

- Movement: Flex your elbows, bringing your chest down and keeping your forearms on the ground. Extend the arms, returning to the plank position.
- Benefit: This variation of push-ups emphasizes the triceps, helping to strengthen the arms and shoulders.

15. BEAR CRAWL (BEAR WALK).

- Starting Position: Stand on all fours, with hands under your shoulders and knees under your hips.
- Movement: Lift your knees off the floor a few inches and walk back and forth, alternately moving your right hand, left foot, and left hand and right foot.
- Benefits: The bear crawl is a fun and challenging exercise that engages the core, arm, and leg muscles, improving coordination and strength.

Remember to perform each exercise with the correct technique and adjust the intensity according to your fitness level. You can create a circuit with these exercises or combine them for a complete training session. Keep varying your routine and experimenting with new activities to keep your workout exciting and motivating. Have a great workout!

5.9 WEEKLY WORKOUT ROUTINES USING FREE-BODY EXERCISES

Each routine focuses on a mix of full-body exercises, with variations in intensity to ensure the right balance between training and recovery. You can start with one way, and as you gain strength and endurance, you can move on to subsequent routines.

ROUTINE 1 - BEGINNER LEVEL

Jumping Jacks - 3 sets x 20 repetitions 1.
2. Push-Ups - 3 sets x 8-10 repetitions
3. Squats - 3 sets x 12-15 repetitions
4. Planks - 3 sets x 30 seconds
5. Glute Bridges - 3 sets x 12-15 repetitions
6. Superman - 3 sets x 10 repetitions
7. Side Plank (both sides) - 3 sets x 20 seconds per side
8. Active rest: Light walking or stretching for 5-10 minutes.

ROUTINE 2 - INTERMEDIATE LEVEL

1. Mountain Climbers - 4 sets x 30 seconds
2. Tricep Dips - 4 sets x 10-12 repetitions
3. Lunges - 4 sets x 12 repetitions per leg

4. Bicycle Crunches - 4 sets x 20 reps per side
5. Bird-Dog - 4 sets x 8 repetitions per side
6. Jump Squats - 4 sets x 12-15 reps.
7. Tricep Push-Ups - 4 sets x 8-10 repetitions
8. Active rest: Walking or light jogging for 10-15 minutes.

ROUTINE 3 - ADVANCED LEVEL

1. Burpees - 5 sets x 10 repetitions
2. Side Plank with Hip Dip (both sides) - 5 sets x 12 reps per side
3. Glute Bridges with one leg raised - 5 sets x 10 reps per leg
4. Bear Crawl - 5 sets x 20 steps back and forth
5. Jumping Lunges - 5 sets x 12 repetitions per leg
6. Spiderman Push-Ups - 5 sets x 10 reps per side
7. V-Up - 5 sets x 12 reps.
8. Active rest: Cycling or light running for 15-20 minutes.

ROUTINE 4 - FULL-BODY CIRCUIT

Jumping Jacks - 3 sets x 30 seconds 1.
2. Push-Ups - 3 sets x 12 repetitions
3. Squats - 3 sets x 15 repetitions
4. Planks - 3 sets x 40 seconds
5. Mountain Climbers - 3 sets x 30 seconds
6. Tricep Dips - 3 sets x 10 repetitions
7. Bicycle Crunches - 3 sets x 20 reps per side
8. Glute Bridges - 3 sets x 15 reps.
9. Active rest: Walking or light running for 10 minutes.

ROUTINE 5 - CORE FOCUS

1. Plank to Push-Up - 4 sets x 8 repetitions
2. Russian Twists - 4 sets x 20 repetitions
3. Hanging Leg Raises (if you have a bar) - 4 sets x 10 repetitions
4. Side Plank Hip Dips (both sides) - 4 sets x 12 reps per side
5. V-Ups - 4 sets x 12 reps.
6. Bird-Dog - 4 sets x 10 reps per side
7. Active rest: walking or biking for 10-15 minutes.

ROUTINE 6 - HIGH-INTENSITY INTERVAL TRAINING (HIIT).

Perform each exercise for 40 seconds, followed by 20 seconds of rest. Complete one round of all activities and repeat for 3-4 sets.
1. Burpees
2. Jump Squats
3. Mountain Climbers
4. Push-Ups
5. Jumping Lunges
6. Plank Jacks (in plank, open and close legs)
7. Tricep Dips
8. High Knees (running on the spot by raising the knees)

ROUTINE 7 - TOTAL BODY STRENGTH

1. Squats - 5 sets x 12 repetitions
2. Push-Ups - 5 sets x 10 repetitions
3. Lunges - 5 sets x 10 reps per leg
4. Glute Bridges with one leg raised - 5 sets x 8 reps per leg
5. Tricep Push-Ups - 5 sets x 8 repetitions
6. Plank - 5 sets x 30 seconds
7. Superman - 5 sets x 8 repetitions
8. Active rest: Walking or stretching for 10 minutes.

ROUTINE 8 - ENDURANCE CHALLENGE

Perform each exercise for 1 minute, without a break between exercises. Complete one round of all activities and repeat for 3-4 sets.
1. jumping jacks
2. Burpees
3. Squats
4. Push-Ups
5. Mountain Climbers
6. Bicycle Crunches
7. Plank
8. Jumping Lunges

Each routine can be performed 2-3 times a week, alternating them to avoid boredom and to ensure a variety of stimulation for the body. Be sure to listen to your body, adjust the intensity according to your fitness level, and give yourself proper recovery between training sessions. Enjoy your workout, and keep striving to reach your fitness goals!

With that, we complete the fifth chapter of our guide. The following section will explore many tasty recipes for incorporating anti-inflammatory foods into your diet. Continue to be curious and committed on your path to a healthier life with less inflammation!

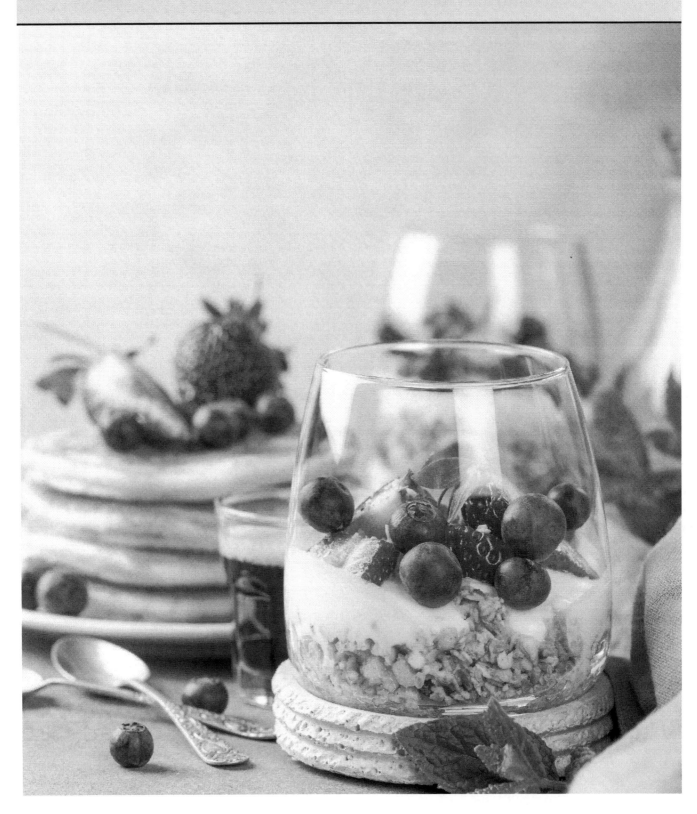

Mushroom Quinoa

Total time: 30 mins / **Prep Time** 10 mins / **Cooking time:** 20 mins / **Difficulty:** Easy

Serving size: 6

Ingredients:

- 1 1/2 pounds of quinoa
- 1 cup of mushrooms
- 1 teaspoon garlic powder
- 3 cloves of garlic, finely chopped
- 1 teaspoon onion powder
- 1 teaspoon Italian seasoning
- salt

Directions:

In a saucepan, place the quinoa and fill flush with water. Add salt and bring to a boil; cook for about 10 minutes. Next, prepare the mushrooms by cutting them fine and placing them in a skillet. Add garlic, onion powder, and Italian seasoning. Cook for about 20 minutes. When done, adjust the salt and stir in the quinoa. Serve hot. You can store it in the refrigerator for up to 7 days.

Nutritional Values: Calories: 145 kcal / Carbohydrates 42g / Protein 28g / Fat 6g / Fiber 13g

Banana Chips

Total time: 100 mins / **Prep Time** 5 mins / **Cooking time:** 90 mins / **Difficulty:** Easy

Serving size: 10

Ingredients:

- 8 bananas, peeled and cut into thin slices
- 1 cup of lemon
- 3 tablespoons lemon juice

Directions:

Set your oven to 255 °F and line a baking sheet with baking paper. In a bowl, mix the water with the lemon juice. Place the sliced bananas on the baking sheet and brush the lemon-water juice on top with a silicone brush. Bake for 90-95 minutes; wait until the bananas become crisp. Also, serve at room temperature.

Nutritional Values: Calories: 90 kcal / Carbohydrates 38g / Protein 12g / Fat 2g / Fiber 18g

Coconut cream pancakes

Total time: 6 hours / **Prep Time** 5 mins / **Cooking time:** 15 mins / **Difficulty:** Easy

Serving size: 6

Ingredients:

For the pancake

- 1 cup of egg whites
- 1/2 cup low-fat yogurt
- 3 tablespoons rice flour
- 3 tablespoons of Coconut Flour Impalpable
- 2 teaspoon Stevia
- 2 teaspoon baking powder
- Water

For the cream

- 1/2 cup of Egg whites
- 1/2 cup approx. of Water
- 6 teaspoons bitter cocoa powder
- 1 banana
- sweetener to taste
- vanilla

For Top

- 2 tablespoons raped coconut

Directions:

In a bowl, whisk the egg and add the yogurt and sweetener. Add the rice flour first and then the coconut flour. Add the baking powder and mix thoroughly. Add a little water and continue mixing. Now pour the mixture into a hot saucepan and turn the heat low. Cook with lid on for about 10 minutes. Cook for another 5 minutes on the other side. Mix the egg white with water, cocoa, vanilla, and the sweetener to prepare the cream. Stir vigorously and cook over low heat, stirring with a kitchen whisk. Now whisk the cooked cream with a ripe banana. When cold, spread the cream over your pancake. Sprinkle with the raped coconut and sit in the refrigerator for at least 6 hours. Serve

Nutritional Values: Calories: 154 kcal / Carbohydrates 32g / Protein 15g / Fat 9g / Fiber 8g

Mayo Salad

Total time: 45 mins / **Prep Time** 10 mins / **Cooking time:** 35 mins / **Difficulty:** Easy

Serving size: 5

Ingredients:

- 3 cups diced potatoes
- 2 cups diced carrots
- 2 cups frozen or fresh peas
- 3 tablespoons oil
- 3 teaspoons vinegar
- pickled gherkins
- 2 cups mayonnaise
- a few leaves of parsley

Directions:

Cook peas in a pot of boiling water. After about 6 minutes, add the potatoes and carrots. After 11 minutes, check that the vegetables are cooked and drain them by placing them in a bowl. In the meantime, prepare the pickled gherkins, and cut them fine. When the vegetables are cold, mix the gherkins with the vegetables. Now add the oil, vinegar, and mayonnaise. Mix everything well. Before serving, add a few parsley leaves, and serve cold.
Nutritional Values: Calories: 157 kcal / Carbohydrates 12g / Protein 8g / Fat 19g / Fiber 13g

Vegetables Quinoa

Total time: 25 mins / **Prep Time** 15 mins / **Cooking time:** 15 mins / **Difficulty:** Easy

Serving size: 8

Ingredients:

- 3 cups of quinoa
- 3 ounces of radicchio
- 1/4 lb. carrots
- 1 stalk of celery
- 1 onion, peeled and finely chopped
- 4 ounces string cheese
- 1 cup cooked and drained spinach
- 1 tablespoon Italian seasoning
- 1 tablespoon onion powder

Directions:

In a saucepan, cook the quinoa and onion with water for about 15 minutes. At the terminus, drain and let drain. Cut the carrots and celery into small cubes in a large bowl, add the finely chopped radicchio, and season with the Italian dressing and onion powder. Stir. Now put the chopped vegetables with the quinoa and add the spinach and d the cheese. Serve warm.
Nutritional Values: Calories: 118 kcal / Carbohydrates 34g / Protein 21g / Fat 7g / Fiber 21g

Bread with alkaline vegetable cream

Total time: 10 mins / **Prep Time** 10 mins / **Cooking time:** / **Difficulty:** Easy

Serving size: 4

Ingredients:

- 2 cups of 5-grain whole-wheat bread
- 2 carrots
- 1 stalk of celery
- a few basil leaves
- 1 avocado
- 1 teaspoon of rosemary powder

Directions:

Wash and dry all the vegetables. Peel the avocado and remove the seed. Put the carrots, celery, and avocado in a blender, add the basil and repeatedly blend for about 1 minute. You should get a thick cream. Add the rosemary powder. Cut your bread into large slices, spread the cream on top, and serve.
Nutritional Values: Calories: 98 kcal / Carbohydrates 27g / Protein 28g / Fat 9g / Fiber 33g

Zucchini Muffin

Total time: 60 mins / **Prep Time** 10 mins / **Cooking time:** 50 mins / **Difficulty:** Easy

Serving size: 8

Ingredients:

- 5 zucchini, peeled and grated
- 1 cup of flour
- 2 eggs

- 1/8 cup sugar
- salt
- 1 teaspoon baking powder

Directions:

In a pan, place zucchini and a drizzle of water, cook for 10 minutes, steamed and with a lid. When done, drain the zucchini and place it in a large bowl. Add the flour with the eggs and baking powder. Give it a quick stir and slowly add the water until you have a smooth dough. Put the mixture into muffin cups and bake in a hot oven at 380°F for about 40 minutes. Serve warm or chilled.

Nutritional Values: Calories: 114 kcal / Carbohydrates 32g / Protein 8g / Fat 11g / Fiber 17g

carrot juice

Total time: 10 mins / **Prep Time** 10 mins / **Cooking time:** / **Difficulty:** Easy

Serving size: 12

Ingredients:

- 15 peeled carrots
- juice of 1 lemon
- 1 kiwi, peeled
- 1 teaspoon sweetener
- 1 teaspoon sweet honey
- a pinch of salt
- mint leaves

Directions:

In a juice extractor, place the roughly chopped carrots and kiwi. Extract the juice and add the lemon juice and sweetener. Stir and add the honey before serving with a pinch of salt. Stir and fill with a few mint leaves and ice if desired.

Nutritional Values: Calories: 81 kcal / Carbohydrates 29g / Protein 12g / Fat 1g / Sugar 11g

Potato Salad

Total time: 20 mins / **Prep Time** 5 mins / **Cooking time:** 15 mins / **Difficulty:** Easy

Serving size: 4

Ingredients:

- 1 head of white cauliflower

- 1/2 head of lettuce
- 1 tablespoon Italian dressing
- 6 medium potatoes, peeled and cut into small cubes.
- Salt
- Oil for seasoning

Directions:

Place water and potatoes with salt in a saucepan. Bring to a boil and cook for about 15 minutes over medium heat. Drain when done. In the meantime, prepare the vegetables by placing cauliflower and lettuce cut to your liking in a bowl. Add the Italian dressing and then the cooked potatoes. Stir and serve cold with a drizzle of oil.

Nutritional Values: Calories: 86 kcal / Carbohydrates 34g / Protein 8g / Fat 3g / Fiber 14g

Banana Porridge

Total time: 20 mins / **Prep Time** 5 mins / **Cooking time:** 15 mins / **Difficulty:** Easy

Serving size: 6

Ingredients:

- 1/4-pound oats
- 1 cup of milk
- 1 tablespoon cinnamon
- 2 bananas
- 1 teaspoon honey

Directions:

In a saucepan, mix the oats with the milk and bring them to a boil. Add the mashed banana, lower the heat, and continue stirring for about 7 minutes. When the mixture thickens, the oatmeal is ready. Serve with a drizzle of honey and a few slices of raw banana.

Nutritional Values: Calories: 102 kcal / Carbohydrates 32g / Protein 19g / Fat 4g / Fiber 22g

Breakfast salad

Total time: 120 mins / **Prep Time** 15 mins / **Cooking time:** / **Difficulty:** Easy

Serving size: 8

Ingredients:

- 1/2 head of green lettuce

- 1/2 head of radicchio
- 1/2 head of white cabbage
- 2 carrots, peeled and cut into rounds
- 1/2 cup corn
- 5 tablespoons shelled and chopped walnuts
- 1 drizzle of corn oil
- 2 tablespoons agave syrup
- salt

Directions:

In a large salad bowl, put the washed vegetables, add the carrots and toss. Now add the corn, nuts, and agave syrup. Store in the refrigerator for about 2 hours. Before serving, add salt and mix.

Nutritional Values: Calories: 97 kcal / Carbohydrates 38g / Protein 8g / Fat 2g / Fiber 38g

Butternut Squash

Total time: 120 mins / **Prep Time** 15 mins / **Cooking time:** / **Difficulty:** Easy

Serving size: 6

Ingredients:

- 1.5 lb. butternut squash, peeled and cut into pieces
- 2 medium parsnips, peeled and cut into pieces
- 2 tbsp. olive oil
- 1 tablespoon chopped fresh sage leaves, plus leaves for garnish
- Salt and black pepper
- Thyme for garnish
- 4 slices of bacon
- 1 onion, thinly sliced
- 1 medium bunch of kale, stemmed and chopped
- 1 tablespoon butter
- 1 tablespoon apple cider vinegar
- 1 c. Gruyere (or Swiss) cheese, cut into pieces
- 2 smoked (or simply toasted) almonds, chopped

Directions:

Preheat the oven to 390°F. Place squash in an ovenproof dish and season with salt, oil, black pepper, parsnips, and thyme. Bake for about 70 minutes and stir every 20 minutes.

Meanwhile, cook the bacon over medium heat in a skillet for about 10 minutes. Crumble it into small pieces and let it cool. Now cook the onions with the cabbage, butter, and vinegar. Add more salt and pepper, and finally, the cooked bacon again. Now mix all the ingredients in the baking dish, trying to keep an even layer. Serve hot.

Nutritional Values: Calories: 118 kcal / Carbohydrates 41g / Protein 12g / Fat 8g / Fiber 29g

Alkaline Minestrone

Total time: 80 mins / **Prep Time** 15 mins / **Cooking time:** 65 mins / **Difficulty:** Easy

Serving size: 5

Ingredients:

- 5 carrots
- 5 potatoes
- 1 celery stalk
- 2 onions, peeled and cut into quarters
- 2 teaspoons garlic powder
- 2 teaspoons onion powder
- 1/4 cup squash
- 4 cherry tomatoes, washed and whole
- Salt

Directions:

In a large saucepan, put all the vegetables and salt- Fill 3/4 full of water and bring to a boil. As soon as it boils, cook for about 60 minutes on low heat. When done, you can eat the detoxifying vegetables individually and reuse the liquid for other recipes.

Nutritional Values: Calories: 59 kcal / Carbohydrates 22g / Protein 9g / Fat 1g / Fiber 44g

Lemon Smoothie

Total time: 10 mins / **Prep Time** 10 mins / **Cooking time:** / **Difficulty:** Easy

Serving size: 6

Ingredients:

- 4 lemons

- 2 apples
- 1 tablespoon eucalyptus honey
- 1 teaspoon stevia, or your favorite sweetener
- a few mint leaves
- a pinch of salt

Directions:

Peel the lemons and save the zest of 1/2 lemon. Grate the zest into a small glass bowl and mix with the salt. Put the lemons and apples in an extractor and wash with the peel. Recover the juice and add the honey and sweetener. Stir. Serve chilled with a few mint leaves and 1 teaspoon of lemon zest per glass. You can add ice as well.

Nutritional Values: Calories: 68 kcal / Carbohydrates 19g / Protein 11g / Fat 0g / Fiber 2g

Cabbage Salad

Total time: 20 mins / **Prep Time** 20 mins / **Cooking time:** / **Difficulty:** Easy

Serving size: 5

Ingredients:

- 1 head of red cabbage
- 2 ounces of vegetable oil
- 5 ounces of red wine vinegar
- sugar
- 3 teaspoons onion powder
- Salt and black pepper

Directions:

Chop one half of the cabbage finely, while the other half chop coarsely and put everything in a bowl. Prepare the dressing by placing the oil, vinegar, sugar, and onion powder in a small bowl. Finally, add the sage and black pepper. Your sauce is ready. Add it to the cabbage and mix. Conserve in the refrigerator for at least a day, so the cabbage will turn redder and release its aromas. Serve cold.

Nutritional Values: Calories: 88 kcal / Carbohydrates 21g / Protein 15g / Fat 1g / Fiber 22g

Red Thai Vegetable curry

Total time: 30 mins / **Prep Time** 10 mins / **Cooking time:** 20 mins / **Difficulty:** Easy

Serving size: 4

Ingredients:

- 2 cups of coconut milk
- 4 tbsp curry paste
- 1 red bell pepper, large
- 1 potato, peeled and cut into pieces
- 1 broccoli
- 1 tablespoon sugar
- 3 tablespoons soy sauce
- 1 ounce of tomato paste
- A few basil leaves

Directions:

Place 10 tablespoons of coconut milk in a saucepan and bring to a boil. Add the red curry paste and stir frequently. Wait until it thickens and add the tomato paste. Cook for about 2 minutes more. Add the rest of the coconut milk and mix it with the soy sauce, sugar, broccoli, and potatoes. Bring your mixture to a boil and lower the heat. Let it simmer for about 15 minutes. Add the bell pepper and continue cooking. Serve with a few basil leaves.

Nutritional Values: Calories: 114 kcal / Carbohydrates 22g / Protein 19g / Fat 6g / Fiber 21g

Zucchini Home Fries

Total time: 20 mins / **Prep Time** 5 mins / **Cooking time:** 15 mins / **Difficulty:** Easy

Serving size: 8

Ingredients:

- 6 large zucchini
- 1/2 cup of breadcrumbs
- a few leaves of parsley, finely chopped
- 1 teaspoon of garlic powder
- 1 teaspoon of Italian seasoning
- 3 eggs
- salt

Directions:

Wash the courgettes and cut them into small sticks. In a bowl, beat the eggs and add the salt. Put the breadcrumbs on a plate, and season with salt, garlic powder, and Italian seasoning. Add the parsley and mix. Now dip the courgettes first in the egg and then in the breadcrumbs and place them in a bowl. In a large pan, put the oil and heat. When hot, add the courgettes and cook them for about 5-7 minutes per side. Wait for them to become crisp and put them to dry on a plate with absorbent paper. Serve hot with your favorite sauce.

Alternatively, use an air fryer to prepare your chips. Cook for 10 minutes at 390 ° F and then for another 5 minutes after turning all the chips in the basket.

Nutritional Values: Calories: 135 kcal / Carbohydrates 29g / Protein 11g / Fat 9g / Fiber 33g

Green Smoothie

Total time: 5 mins / **Prep Time** 5 mins / **Cooking time:** / **Difficulty:** Easy

Serving size: 4

Ingredients:

- 4 kiwis
- 1 banana
- 1/2 cup of white grapes
- 1 teaspoon of honey
- 1 teaspoon of Stevia sweetener
- A few mint leaves
- 1 tablespoon of lemon juice
- salt

Directions:

Put the peeled kiwis, banana, and grapes in a food

extractor. Collect the juice and add the mint and lemon. Stir, and before serving, add a pinch of salt (to taste).

Nutritional Values: Calories: 56 kcal / Carbohydrates 18g / Protein 13g / Fat 1g / Fiber 38g

Hemp Seed Porridge

Total time: 10 mins / **Prep Time** 5 mins / **Cooking time:** 5 mins / **Difficulty:** Easy

Serving size: 8

Ingredients:

- 8 cups of almond milk
- 4 cups of hemp seeds, shelled
- 8 cups of chia seeds
- 3 cups of artisan honey
- 1 cup of flaked almonds.
- 1 cup of flaxseed flour
- salt

Directions:

Mix the almond milk with the chia seeds, flaxseed flour, and honey in a bowl. Add the salt and mix. Now pour the contents into a saucepan and bring to a boil. Cook over low heat and continue stirring until it thickens. Serve in a large bowl and season with flaked almonds.

Nutritional Values: Calories: 112 kcal / Carbohydrates 29g / Protein 23g / Fat 5g / Fiber 6g

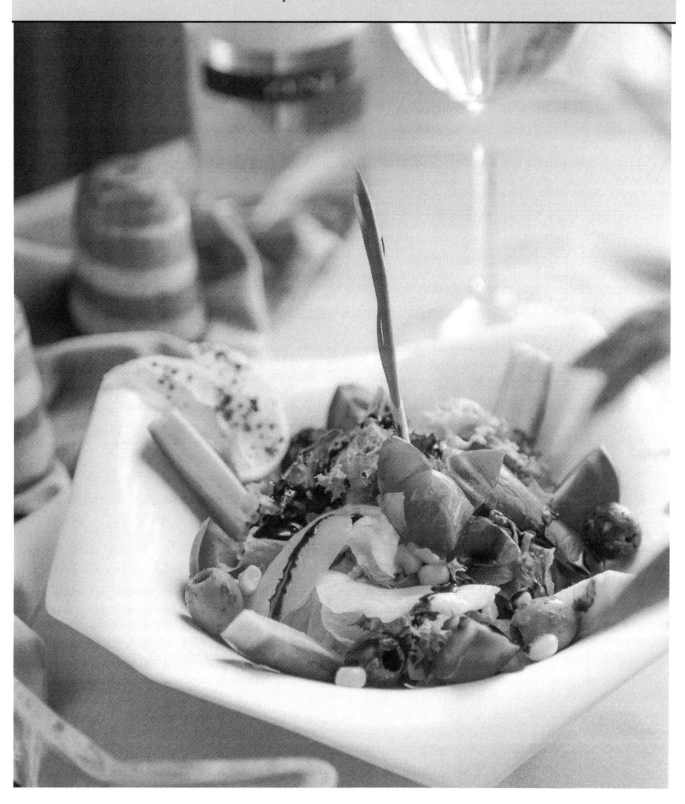

Roasted Tofu with coconut Milk

Total time: 40 mins / **Prep Time** 10 mins / **Cooking time:** 30 mins / **Difficulty:** Easy

Serving size: 6

Ingredients:

- 2 cups of diced tofu
- 3 cups of coconut milk
- 1/2 onion cut into thin slices
- 1 teaspoon of garlic powder
- 1 teaspoon of Italian dressing
- 1 teaspoon of onion powder
- 1 teaspoon of cornstarch
- Salt to taste

Directions:

In a pan, cook the tofu with the onion. Meanwhile, put the coconut milk in a saucepan and mix it with the starch. Start heating, and don't bring it to a boil. Wait for it to thicken, and then add the cream to the roasted tofu. Drizzle with the onion and garlic powder, and add the Italian dressing and salt

Nutritional Values: Calories: 113 kcal / Carbohydrates 40g / Protein 19g / Fat 38g / Fiber 5g

Sweet and Sour Potatoes with Meat

Total time: 50 mins / **Prep Time** 10 mins / **Cooking time:** 40 mins / **Difficulty:** Easy

Serving size: 4

Ingredients:

- 4 slices of veal
- 2 cups of potatoes
- 2 ounces of black olives without seeds
- 2 tablespoons of rosemary leaves
- 1 tablespoon of oil
- 1 teaspoon of Italian dressing

Directions:

Cook the meat in your air fryer, set 390 ° F for 15 minutes, and then for another 5 minutes on the other side. Meanwhile, prepare the potatoes, cut them into large cubes, and place them in a pan. Add the rosemary and a drizzle of oil. Bake in the oven for about 30 minutes. In the end, add the olives and the Italian dressing. Now add the potatoes to the meat and serve hot.

Nutritional Values: Calories: 118 kcal / Carbohydrates 12g / Protein 44g / Fat 19g / Fiber 2g

Stuffed Peppers

Total time: 60 mins / **Prep Time** 10 mins / **Cooking time:** 50 mins / **Difficulty:** Easy

Serving size: 8

Ingredients:

- 2 yellow peppers
- 2 red peppers
- 4 green peppers
- 2 cups of breadcrumbs
- 1/2 head of white cabbage, blanched and soft
- parsley, abundant
- 8 cloves of garlic, finely chopped
- 1 onion, finely chopped
- 1 tablespoon of capers
- 1 pinch of hot pepper
- 1 cup Gruyere cheese, cut into cubes
- salt
- a splash of oil

Directions:

The oven to 385 ° F and line a baking sheet with parchment paper. Wash the peppers and remove the green stalk and the internal seeds. Try to keep the pepper whole. Put the breadcrumbs in a separate bowl, season it with the garlic and onion, and add the capers and, if desired, the hot pepper. With a blender, blend the cauliflower and add it to the crumb. In the end, add the cheese and mix well to mix the ingredients. Using a spoon, pour the crumb inside the peppers and, when complete, compact and close the upper end with a small aluminum foil. Bake for about 45-50 minutes. Before serving, add a drizzle of oil.

Nutritional Values: Calories: 112 kcal / Carbohydrates 33g / Protein 9g / Fat 8g / Fiber 32g

Baked Fish

Total time: 55 mins / **Prep Time** 15 mins / **Cooking time:** 40 mins / **Difficulty:** Easy

Serving size: 4

Ingredients:

- 4 large slices of salmon
- 1 lemon, squeezed
- 4 tablespoons of oil
- salt
- 1 tablespoon of rosemary leaves

Directions:

Set your oven to 390 ° F and line a baking sheet with parchment paper. Mix the lemon juice with the oil and a pinch of salt in a bowl. If you wish, you can also grate the lemon zest inside for a more intense flavor. Add the salmon slices and brush with the prepared dressing. Bake for 35-40 minutes and wait for the salmon to become crisp and well cooked. Just before turning off the oven, add the rosemary and serve hot.
Nutritional Values: Calories: 99 kcal / Carbohydrates 12g / Protein 38g / Fat 31g / Fiber 3g

Onion Omelette

Total time: 25 mins / **Prep Time** 5 mins / **Cooking time:** 20 mins / **Difficulty:** Easy

Serving size: 6

Ingredients:

- 7 large eggs
- 1 teaspoon of garlic powder
- 1 teaspoon of onion powder
- 2 green onions, thinly sliced
- 1/2 cup soft cheese, Leerdammer
- 1 mozzarella, drained

Directions:

In a pan, put the onion and a drizzle of water, and cook over medium heat with a lid for 2-3 minutes; in this way, the onion becomes soft. While the onion is cooking, in a medium bowl, beat the eggs in and add garlic, onion powder, and salt. Start mixing vigorously. In a second bowl, prepare the cheeses by cutting them into cubes. When the onion is ready, add the liquid egg to the pan and the cheeses. Lower the heat slightly and cook for about 10 minutes on each side. Serve hot and stringy.
Nutritional Values: Calories: 115 kcal / Carbohydrates 18g / Protein 41g / Fat 38g / Fiber 9g

Chickpeas and vegetables

Total time: 10 hours / **Prep Time** 20 mins / **Cooking time:** 60 mins / **Difficulty:** Easy

Serving size: 5

Ingredients:

- 2 cups of dried chickpeas
- 1 pinch of baking soda
- 3 carrots
- 1 stalk of celery
- 1 head of cauliflower tops
- 4 tomatoes, quartered
- 1/2 onion, thinly sliced
- 1 tablespoon of tomato concentrate
- 1 teaspoon of Italian dressing
- salt and black pepper

Directions:

In a large bowl, soak the chickpeas with the baking soda and let them sprout overnight. In the end, drain and set aside. Fill a saucepan 3/4 full of water, add the carrots cut into strips, the cauliflower, and the celery. Add the chickpeas with the tomatoes and onion and bring to a boil. Cook for about 60 minutes or until the chickpeas are soft. When cooking is almost done, add the seasonings and season with salt. Serve hot.
Nutritional Values: Calories: 95 kcal / Carbohydrates 24g / Protein 39g / Fat 11g / Fiber 22g

Boiled Chicken

Total time: 35 mins / **Prep Time** 5 mins / **Cooking time:** 30 mins / **Difficulty:** Easy

Serving size: 5

Ingredients:

- 5 slices of chicken breast
- 1 tablespoon of parsley
- 1 teaspoon of garlic powder
- Juice of 1 lemon
- 3 tablespoons of raw oil
- salt

Directions:

In a pan, place the chicken slices with the parsley. Add a drizzle of water and salt and cook with the lid on for about 15 minutes. After the time has elapsed, turn the slices and cook for another 15 minutes, always with a lid. While the chicken is cooking, make the dressing by mixing the lemon juice with oil, salt, and garlic powder. When the chicken is well cooked, place it on the plate and add the prepared dressing. Serve hot.

Nutritional Values: Calories: 91 kcal / Carbohydrates 9g / Protein 37g / Fat 5g / Fiber 1g

Veal with mango sauce

Total time: 50 mins / **Prep Time** 10 mins / **Cooking time:** 20 mins / **Difficulty:** Easy

Serving size: 4

Ingredients:

- 2 mangoes
- 1 apple
- 4 slices of veal without fat
- 1/4 cup black balsamic vinegar
- 1 tablespoon of soy sauce
- 1 teaspoon of garlic powder
- salt

Directions:

In an immersion blender, prepare the sauce by putting the mango and apple. Blend until you get a thick mixture. Add the soy sauce with the vinegar and mix with the garlic powder. The dressing is ready. Now cook the meat for about 20 minutes in a pan and add a pinch of salt if you wish. When the heart is glad, mix it with the prepared sauce and serve it with whole meal bread.

Nutritional Values: Calories: 115 kcal / Carbohydrates 8g / Protein 44g / Fat 11g / Fiber 6g

Baked Tomatoes

Total time: 60 mins / **Prep Time** 10 mins / **Cooking time:** 50 mins / **Difficulty:** Easy

Serving size: 8

Ingredients:

- 10 large tomatoes
- 6 ounces of cubby Leerdammer cheese
- 1 cup of breadcrumbs
- parsley
- salt
- black pepper
- 1 tablespoon of oregano
- 3 tablespoons of rosemary leaves
- a drizzle of raw oil

Directions:

Set your oven to 375 ° F and place the parchment on a baking sheet. Wash your tomato and cut it into quarters. In a bowl, prepare the breadcrumbs and season with salt, parsley, and black pepper. Now pour the breadcrumbs over the tomato and add the oregano and rosemary. Before baking, put the cheese on top and cook for 40-50 minutes. When the cheese is well browned, serve with a drizzle of oil.

Nutritional Values: Calories: 85 kcal / Carbohydrates 12g / Protein 8g / Fat 11g / Fiber 12g

Vegetable Hash

Total time: 40 mins / **Prep Time** 10 mins / **Cooking time:** 30 mins / **Difficulty:** Easy

Serving size: 6

Ingredients:

- 2 eggplants, cut into cubes
- 4 courgettes, cut into cubes
- red pepper, without stalk and seeds
- potatoes, cut into cubes
- 2 large eggs
- 1 teaspoon of garlic powder
- 1 teaspoon of onion powder

- 2 tablespoons of chives

- a few leaves of parsley

- salt

Directions:

In a large saucepan, cook the aubergines with the courgettes over medium heat. Meanwhile, cut the pepper into strips and then add it to the pan with the potatoes. Next, add the garlic and onion powder and mix. Finally, add the chives with the parsley and continue mixing. Cook for about 30 minutes and season with salt. When the vegetables are well cooked, break 2 eggs on top and put a lid on. Cook for about 3-4 minutes. You can add a pinch of black pepper to the eggs if you wish. Serve hot.

Nutritional Values: Calories: 98 kcal / Carbohydrates 16g / Protein 14g / Fat 8g / Fiber 22g

Champignon Omelette

Total time: 50 mins / **Prep Time** 15 mins / **Cooking time:** 35 mins / **Difficulty:** Easy

Serving size: 4

Ingredients:

- 1 cup of champignon mushrooms, washed

- 1/2 onion, finely chopped

- 1 teaspoon of Italian dressing

- 3 cloves of garlic, finely chopped

- chives

- 1 ounce of butter

- a few leaves of parsley

- salt

- 5 large eggs

- 1/2 cup of stringy cheese

Directions:

Cut the mushrooms into small slices. Now put the butter in the pan and add the mushrooms with the garlic. Cook over medium heat for a few minutes, add the onion and chives and stir occasionally. While the mushrooms are cooking, prepare the eggs by beating them in a bowl, and add the cheese and parsley. Add the Italian dressing. Stir and pour directly into the pan. Lower the heat and cook for about 30 minutes. Turn halfway through cooking.

Nutritional Values: Calories: 104 kcal / Carbohydrates 9g / Protein 21g / Fat 24g / Fiber 19g

Chicken with Sweet Potatoes

Total time: 55 mins / **Prep Time** 10 mins / **Cooking time:** 45 mins / **Difficulty:** Easy

Serving size: 6

Ingredients:

- 1 large boneless whole chicken

- 4 potatoes, peeled and cut into large cubes

- 2 tablespoons of sweet and sour sauce

- 1 tablespoon of rosemary

- 1 teaspoon of Italian dressing

- black pepper

- 1/2 cup of soft cheese

- salt

Directions:

Preheat your oven to 390 ° F and line a baking sheet with parchment paper. Place the chicken on top and toss it with the Italian dressing and cheese. Now add the potatoes and bake. Cook for about 20-25 minutes. Now add the sweet and sour sauce and rosemary, finish with salt and black pepper and bake for another 20 minutes or so. The chicken should be well cooked and soft. Serve hot.

Nutritional Values: Calories: 115 kcal / Carbohydrates 14g / Protein 33g / Fat 19g / Fiber 7g

Mix Grilled Vegetables

Total time: 6 hours / **Prep Time** 15 mins / **Cooking time:** 35 mins / **Difficulty:** Easy

Serving size: 5

Ingredients:

- 1 red pepper

- 1 yellow pepper

- 1 eggplant, peeled

- 2 courgettes, peeled and cut into rings

- 3 carrots, peeled and cut into rings

- 1 onion, cut into thick slices

- 3 tablespoons of citrus sauce for seasoning

Directions:

Cut the eggplant into round slices and soak them in a bowl with water and salt overnight. Make sure they are all immersed in the liquid. Cut the peppers into strips and remove the seeds and the green stalk. Drain the aubergines and put them in a bowl with the other vegetables. Prepare your grill and start heating. When hot, place the vegetables and cook for about 15 minutes per side. When they're almost ready, sprinkle your favorite sauce on top. Serve hot.

Alternatively, you can prepare this recipe using the air fryer, setting the temperature to 390 ° F. Cook for 15-20 minutes on each side.

Nutritional Values: Calories: 82 kcal / Carbohydrates 24g / Protein 19g / Fat 4g / Fiber 41g

Vegetables and Lentils

Total time: 60 mins / **Prep Time** 20 mins / **Cooking time:** 40 mins / **Difficulty:** Easy

Serving size: 5

Ingredients:

- 2 cups of lentils
- 1 stalk of celery
- 1 carrot, peeled and cut into 1-inch pieces
- 1 head of cauliflower, pureed
- 1/2 head of radicchio
- 3 ounces of cooked corn
- 1 cooked turnip
- raw oil
- salt
- 1 teaspoon of Italian dressing
- 2 tsp chives

Directions:

I n a saucepan, cook the lentils with water and salt. Add the celery and carrot. Bring to a boil and cook for about 35-40 minutes. In a salad bowl, prepare the other vegetables, adding cauliflower, radicchio, and corn. Stir and add the turnip. When the lentils are well cooked, add them to the vegetables, season with salt, and add the Italian dressing and chives. Serve.

Nutritional Values: Calories: 93 kcal / Carbohydrates 33g / Protein 42g / Fat 5g / Fiber 44g

Artichokes and quinoa

Total time: 25 mins / **Prep Time** 5 mins / **Cooking time:** 20 mins / **Difficulty:** Easy

Serving size: 8

Ingredients:

- 2 and a half pounds of quinoa
- 12 artichoke hearts in oil
- 1/2 head of cauliflower tops
- 4 ounces of soft cheese, cut into cubes
- 2 tablespoons of chives
- Salt and black pepper for seasoning

Directions:

Rinse the quinoa in a colander with cold water. Put the drained quinoa in a saucepan and fill it with water. Add the salt and bring it to a boil. Cook for about 15-20 minutes and then drain again. Put the quinoa in a bowl and add artichokes. Add the chives and cauliflower. Top with the cheese and mix so that it melts. Season with salt and black pepper and serve hot.

Nutritional Values: Calories: 88 kcal / Carbohydrates 41g / Protein 22g / Fat 9g / Fiber 26g

Stuffed Eggplant

Total time: 65 mins / **Prep Time** 15 mins / **Cooking time:** 50 mins / **Difficulty:** Easy

Serving size: 6

Ingredients:

- 6 large eggplants
- 1 cup of crumb
- a few leaves of parsley
- 1 tablespoon of garlic powder
- 1 tablespoon of onion powder
- 1 ounce of chives
- 1 head of cauliflower, pureed
- chili pepper to taste
- salt and black pepper in granules

Directions:

Peel the aubergines and cut them into thin slices. In a bowl, prepare the dressing, putting the breadcrumbs and adding the parsley and chives. Next, add the salt and garlic, and onion powder. Stir and finally add the pureed cauliflower. Preheat the oven to 380 ° F and prepare a large baking sheet with parchment paper. Arrange the aubergines and add the seasoning on top of each slice. If you wish, add the chili and black pepper in granules. Cook for 40-50 minutes, ensuring the eggplant is well cooked. If they are still raw, increase to 395 ° F and cook for another 10-15 minutes. **Nutritional Values:** Calories: 92 kcal / Carbohydrates 38g / Protein 15g / Fat 8g / Fiber 33g

Baked Onions and Potatoes

Total time: 50 mins / **Prep Time** 10 mins / **Cooking time:** 40 mins / **Difficulty:** Easy

Serving size: 9

Ingredients:

- 2 cups of potatoes
- 1 pound of onions, cut into 8 parts each
- 2 cups of couscous
- 1 tablespoon of garlic powder
- 1 tablespoon of onion powder
- 2 tablespoons of rosemary
- raw oil
- salt and black pepper

Directions:

Peel the potatoes and cut them into cubes. Place the potatoes with onions in a baking tray lined with a paper oven and bake in a preheated oven at 380 ° F for 40 minutes. Meanwhile, prepare the couscous by filling a saucepan 1/2 cup with water and salt and bring to a boil. When it boils, pour in the couscous and turn off the heat. Let it rest for about 30 minutes. When done, add the garlic and onion powder and drizzle with a bit of oil. When the potatoes are ready, add the rosemary and black pepper to taste. Season with salt according to taste. Stir in the couscous and serve hot. **Nutritional Values:** Calories: 96 kcal / Carbohydrates 42g / Protein 18g / Fat 6g / Fiber 29g

Spicy Meat

Total time: 30 mins / **Prep Time** 10 mins / **Cooking time:** 20 mins / **Difficulty:** Easy

Serving size: 4

Ingredients:

- 4 slices of pork
- 2 tablespoons of hot sauce
- 1 teaspoon of chives
- a drizzle of oil
- 1 teaspoon of garlic powder
- 1 teaspoon of Italian dressing
- 1/2 onion, finely chopped

Directions:

In a skillet, cook the meat with the onion. Roast for about 10 minutes on each side. As you cook the meat, prepare the dressing in a bowl by placing the hot sauce and mixing it with the chives, garlic powder, and Italian dressing. When the heart is ready, add the seasoning on top. Season with salt to taste and serve hot. **Nutritional Values:** Calories: 98 kcal / Carbohydrates 12g / Protein 44g / Fat 12g / Fiber 5g

Mix Fermented Vegetables

Total time: 10 mins / **Prep Time** 10 mins / **Cooking time:** / **Difficulty:** Easy

Serving size: 6

Ingredients:

- 1 head of cauliflower, pureed
- 1/2 bunch of green lettuce
- 2 tablespoons of fermented artichokes
- 2 tablespoons of fermented zucchini
- 2 tablespoons of fermented cucumber
- 2 tablespoons of fermented corn
- 1 tablespoon of rosemary
- 1 drizzle of oil
- Salt

Directions:

Fermented foods contain many friendly bacteria and help digestive processes. Take all the fermented vegetables and put them in a bowl. Add a drizzle of oil and rosemary and mix. Add the cauliflower and green lettuce. Season with a sauce to your liking and season with salt. Serve cool.

Nutritional Values: Calories: 75 kcal / Carbohydrates 14g / Protein 18g / Fat 1g / Fiber 22g

Asparagus Omelette

Total time: 30 mins / **Prep Time** 10 mins / **Cooking time:** 20 mins / **Difficulty:** Easy

Serving size: 3

Ingredients:

- 4 large eggs
- 1/2 cup of milk
- 1 ounce of stringy cheese
- black pepper
- 2 bunches of asparagus without stem
- 1/2 onion
- 1 ounce of butter
- salt

Directions:

In a pan, melt the butter and sauté the onion quickly. Add the asparagus and cook for a few minutes. Meanwhile, prepare the eggs by beating them in a bowl with milk and cheese. Combine with black pepper and pour the liquid egg into the pan when the onions are ready. Cook for 10 minutes on each side. Serve hot.

Nutritional Values: Calories: 96 kcal / Carbohydrates 12g / Protein 29g / Fat 19g / Fiber 3g

Roasted Eggplant

Total time: 10 hours / **Prep Time** 10 mins / **Cooking time:** 35 mins / **Difficulty:** Easy

Serving size: 10

Ingredients:

- 3 large eggplants
- salt
- thyme
- 1 teaspoon of onion powder
- 1 teaspoon of garlic powder
- 2 ounces of raw oil
- parsley

Directions:

Peel the aubergines and cut them into large, not too thick, slices. In a large bowl, put the aubergines and fill them with water, thyme, and salt. Soak them for at least 10 hours. When done, drain and prepare your grill. When hot, add the aubergines, cook them for 15-20 minutes per side, and ensure they are well cooked. When finished, put your aubergines in a bowl, season them with the onion and garlic powder, and add the parsley with the oil. Serve hot.

Nutritional Values: Calories: 79 kcal / Carbohydrates 22g / Protein 17g / Fat 3g / Fiber 39g

CHAPTER 8: DINNER RECIPES

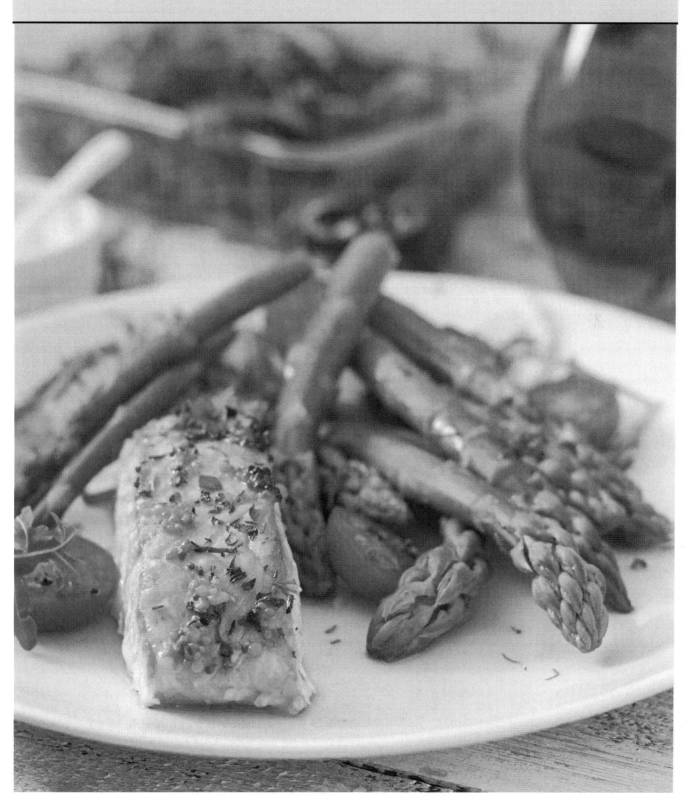

Cilantro lime quinoa

Total time: 15 mins / **Prep Time** 5 mins / **Cooking time:** 10 mins / **Difficulty:** Easy

Serving size: 8

Ingredients:

- meat hash
- 3 cups of whole meal Quinoa
- 1 lime
- a few leaves of cilantro
- 1 drizzle of oil
- 1 tablespoon of turmeric
- 1 tablespoon of curry
- salt

Directions:

In a saucepan, put the water and salt and bring to a boil. When it boils, add the Quinoa and cook over low heat for about 10 minutes. When it is ready, drain and let it rest. In a bowl, prepare the dressing by putting the cilantro leaves and mixing them with the turmeric and curry. Add the Quinoa and continue mixing. Drizzle with a drizzle of oil and serve hot.

Nutritional Values: Calories: 95 kcal / Carbohydrates 29g / Protein 22g / Fat 2g / Fiber 29g

Spinach Quinoa

Total time: 35 mins / **Prep Time** 15 mins / **Cooking time:** 20 mins / **Difficulty:** Easy

Serving size: 8

Ingredients:

- 3 cups of rice
- 1 pound of asparagus
- 1 onion, peeled and thinly sliced
- 1 small potato, peeled and thinly sliced
- 2 tablespoons of white wine
- 3 tablespoons of butter
- 1 teaspoon of onion powder
- 1 teaspoon of Italian dressing.

- salt
- 2 tablespoons of Parmesan cheese, grated

Directions:

Prepare the asparagus by washing them and taking the tips. In a large skillet, sauté the onion and butter quickly. When the onion starts to brown, add the asparagus and the potato. Cook for a few minutes, stirring frequently. Try to mix all the ingredients. Now add a small amount of water and the rice. Lower the heat and stir often. When the risotto dries, you must add a small amount of water and continue stirring. Repeat these steps until the rice is soft, then cook for about 45 minutes, stirring frequently. When you are almost done cooking, add the onion powder and the Italian seasoning and mix. When the rice is almost ready, add the white wine and the Parmesan cheese and season with salt. Finally, you choose the consistency of your risotto by continuing to cook. Serve hot with half-cooked asparagus or two on the plate.

Nutritional Values: Calories: 102 kcal / Carbohydrates 38g / Protein 12g / Fat 11g / Fiber 9g

Pineapple and Carrot Salad

Total time: 15 mins / **Prep Time** 15 mins / **Cooking time:** / **Difficulty:** Easy

Serving size: 5

Ingredients:

- 1 pineapple, peeled and sliced
- 4 peeled carrots
- juice of half a lemon
- 1 tablespoon of chestnut honey, liquid
- 2 tablespoons of maple syrup
- 1 pinch of salt (to taste)

Directions:

In a large bowl, cut the pineapple into small pieces. Next, cut 3 carrots into slices, the last grater. Mix the carrots with the pineapple and add the honey. Mix the maple syrup with the lemon juice in a small bowl, add the salt, and mix. Pour it over the pineapple and mix everything. Serve cold.

Nutritional Values: Calories: 88 kcal / Carbohydrates 41g / Protein 3g / Fat 2g / Fiber 24g

Peppers Pizza

Total time: 75 mins / **Prep Time** 15 mins /
Cooking time: 60 mins / **Difficulty:** Easy

Serving size: 3

Ingredients:

- 1 cup of flour
- 1 cube of fresh yeast
- salt
- 1 green pepper
- 1 yellow pepper
- 1/2 onion
- 1/2 onion
- 1 cup of soft cheese, grated
- 1/2 cup cooked tomato sauce

Directions:

In a large bowl, put the flour, salt, and yeast. Gradually add the water and start kneading with your hands. Try to get a thick and non-sticky dough. Alternatively, you can use your mixer and follow the directions. Transfer the dough to a bowl and let it rise for about 1 hour or until it doubles in size. Meanwhile, prepare the dressing, cut the peppers into thin strips, remove the seeds and mix them with the finely chopped onion. When the dough has risen, make 3 loaves and roll out each one with the help of a rolling pin. Put the sauce first, then the cheese, and finally the peppers and onion. Bake at 400 ° F for 40-50 minutes, until the dough is well cooked and leavened. Serve hot.
Nutritional Values: Calories: 118 kcal / Carbohydrates 32g / Protein 12g / Fat 7g / Fiber 19g

Healthy Broccoli and Asparagus

Total time: 25 mins / **Prep Time** 5 mins /
Cooking time: 20 mins / **Difficulty:** Easy

Serving size: 6

Ingredients:

- 1 large broccoli
- 1 bunch of asparagus (about 1 cup)
- 2 carrots, peeled and grated
- 1 lemon
- salt

Directions:

Wash your vegetables, peel the broccoli and take the tops. Next, cut the tips of the asparagus and discard the stem.
In a saucepan, put a drizzle of water and salt and bring to a boil. Pour in the broccoli and asparagus, lower the heat and cook with the lid on for 15-20 minutes. During cooking, ensure there is always a trickle of water to maintain the steam. When cooked, put them in a bowl, and add the grated carrots and lemon; you can also grate and squeeze them if you wish. Season with salt and serve cool.
Nutritional Values: Calories: 76 kcal / Carbohydrates 28g / Protein 14g / Fat 1g / Fiber 39g

Baked Pumpkin

Total time: 5 mins / **Prep Time** 5 mins / **Cooking time:** 40 mins / **Difficulty:** Easy

Serving size: 7

Ingredients:

- 1 large pumpkin
- 1 tablespoon of onion powder
- 1 tablespoon of Italian dressing
- 1/4 cup of vinegar
- black pepper for seasoning
- salt

Directions:

Peel your pumpkin, cut it in half and remove the internal seeds. Continue dividing the pumpkin until it forms small slices; now, miss it like chips. Preheat the oven to 380 ° F and line a pan with parchment paper. Place the chopped pumpkin on top and pour a part of black pepper, the onion powder, and the Italian seasoning over each slice. Give a sprinkle of vinegar and add salt to taste. Cook for about 40 minutes until the squash is well done. Serve at room temperature.
Nutritional Values: Calories: 84 kcal / Carbohydrates 39g / Protein 8g / Fat 2g / Fiber 33g

Pumpkin Risotto

Total time: 80 mins / **Prep Time** 20 mins /
Cooking time: 60 mins / **Difficulty:** Easy

Serving size: 12

Ingredients:

- 1 giant pumpkin, peeled and diced, without seeds,
- 3 cups of rice for risotto
- 1 white onion, peeled and sliced
- 2 ounces of butter
- 1 teaspoon of garlic powder
- 1 teaspoon of onion powder
- 1 glass (1/4 cup approximately) of white wine
- salt
- A few thyme leaves to decorate

Directions:

In a large pan, sauté the onion, butter, and salt quickly. As soon as the onion starts to brown, add the pumpkin and mix to blend the ingredients. After a few minutes, add the water, wait for it to boil, and add the rice. Make sure your mixture is always well hydrated and mixed. Cook for about 40 minutes, add the onion and garlic powder, season with salt, and cook for another 20 minutes. When you are almost at the end of cooking, add the white wine to further flavor, let it thicken, and turn off the heat when the risotto reaches the consistency you prefer. Serve hot on a plate with a few thyme leaves.

Nutritional Values: Calories: 112 kcal / Carbohydrates 41g / Protein 12g / Fat 15g / Fiber 9g

Mixed Legumes Soup

Total time: 10 hours / **Prep Time** 10 mins / **Cooking time:** 75 mins / **Difficulty:** Easy

Serving size: 4

Ingredients:

- 1/2 onion
- 1/2 cup of dry beans
- 1/2 cup of dried chickpeas
- 1/2 cup of lentils
- 4 tomatoes, washed and quartered
- 2 carrots, peeled and cut into rings
- 1 stalk of celery
- 1 teaspoon of onion powder

- 1 teaspoon of garlic powder
- 1 teaspoon of curry
- a few leaves of thyme
- 1 teaspoon of baking soda
- salt

Directions:

Soak the beans and chickpeas in a large bowl overnight and add a teaspoon of baking soda. Drain and transfer to a saucepan. Add the lentils and onion. Fill with water and add the tomatoes, carrots, and celery. Bring to a boil and cook for about 70-75 minutes, stirring occasionally. When you are finished cooking, add the onion and garlic powder, and before serving, add a few leaves of thyme and season with salt. Serve hot.

Nutritional Values: Calories: 100 kcal / Carbohydrates 38g / Protein 45g / Fat 3g / Fiber 29g

Zucchini Risotto

Total time: 45 mins / **Prep Time** 10 mins / **Cooking time:** 35 mins / **Difficulty:** Easy

Serving size: 6

Ingredients:

- 2 pounds of brown rice
- 4 courgettes, peeled and cut into rings
- 2 ounces of butter
- 1 soft cheese, Leerdammer (or similar)
- 1 vegetable cube, homemade
- 1 glass of white wine
- 1/2 white onion, thinly sliced
- salt to taste
- 2 bay leaves

Directions:

In a large skillet, put the zucchini and onion. Add the butter and heat. When the onions start to brown, add the rice and stir for 1 minute. Add the water slowly and continue stirring; you need to get a very light boil. Cook for 30-35 minutes until it becomes the density you want. After about 20 minutes, add the nut and bay leaf. When you are done cooking, add the cheese and wine. Cook briefly for 1 minute. Serve hot

Nutritional Values: Calories: 122 kcal /

Carbohydrates 42g / Protein 13g / Fat 11g / Fiber 8g

Pineapple and Coconut

Total time: 10 mins / **Prep Time** 10 mins / **Cooking time:** / **Difficulty:** Easy

Serving size: 6

Ingredients:

- 1 large pineapple, peeled
- 1 coconut, peeled and without the brown skin
- 1 cup of coconut milk
- 1 ounce of ginger
- 12 slices of whole meal bread, rustic

Directions:

Cut the pineapple into slices in a large bowl and add 1-inch-sized chopped coconut pieces. Add the milk and mix. Grate over the ginger and give it a quick stir. For each serving, place 2 wet slices of bread in the bowl and then on the plate. And put the remaining liquid on the other side of the container. Serve cold

Nutritional Values: Calories: 144 kcal / Carbohydrates 29g / Protein 18g / Fat 24g / Fiber 22g

Chicken Muffin

Total time: 55 mins / **Prep Time** 10 mins / **Cooking time:** 45 mins / **Difficulty:** Easy

Serving size: 10

Ingredients:

- 1/2 chicken, boneless
- 1 cup of flour
- 1 teaspoon of yeast
- 1/2 onion
- 1 teaspoon of Italian dressing
- 3 tablespoons of seed oil
- salt
- 3 eggs

Directions:

Add the chicken and onion to a saucepan with a drizzle of water. Cook with the lid on for about 10-15 minutes until the meat is tender and white. Put the chicken and onion in a blender, add the Italian dressing and oil, and blend. Try to get a homogeneous mixture. Now prepare the muffins by putting the flour and baking powder in a bowl and add a drizzle of salt and the eggs. Start kneading, and then add the smoothie chicken. Knead until you get a homogeneous and dense mixture. Now pour the mixture into muffin cups and bake in your oven at 395 ° F for about 30 minutes. Serve hot

Nutritional Values: Calories: 98 kcal / Carbohydrates 38g / Protein 28g / Fat 11g / Fiber 2g

Raw Rainbow Vegetables

Total time: 10 mins / **Prep Time** 10 mins / **Cooking time:** / **Difficulty:** Easy

Serving size: 8

Ingredients:

- 1 head of white cabbage
- 1 head of broccoli,
- 4 carrots, peeled
- 1 head of radicchio
- 1 head of green lettuce, soft
- 1 ounce of palm oil, raw
- salt
- 1/2 cup of Greek yogurt
- 1 teaspoon of garlic powder
- 1 lemon, cut into small slices

Directions:

In a large salad bowl, put the pureed cabbage, and the carrots cut into rings. Next, add only the broccoli tops and the washed radicchio. Finish by adding the washed and cut small green lettuce leaves. In a second bowl, mix the yogurt with oil and the garlic powder, add the juice of half a lemon, and mix. Season your salad, and you can add the remaining lemon to your rainbow salad. Serve fresh.

Nutritional Values: Calories: 86 kcal / Carbohydrates 36g / Protein 11g / Fat 3g / Fiber 46g

Fresh fruit and Vanilla

Total time: 15 mins / **Prep Time** 15 mins / **Cooking time:** / **Difficulty:** Easy

Serving size: 5

Ingredients:

- 1 avocado, peeled and seeded
- 1 mango
- 1 banana, roughly chopped
- 1 apple, peeled and quartered
- 2 kiwifruit, peeled and cut into 4 parts
- 2 tablespoons of maple syrup
- 1 tablespoon of honey
- 1/4 cup of pureed walnuts
- 3 ounces of vanilla-flavored plain yogurt
- 1 pinch of salt

Directions:

In a large salad bowl, place your coarsely chopped fruit. Add the maple syrup and walnuts. Mix by adding the yogurt and honey. If you wish, you can also add salt to enhance the flavors. Keep in the fridge for 1 hour before serving.

Nutritional Values: Calories: 110 kcal / Carbohydrates 38g / Protein 3g / Fat 2g / Fiber 44g

Vegetables with green toppings

Total time: 25 mins / **Prep Time** 25 mins / **Cooking time:** / **Difficulty:** Easy

Serving size: 7

Ingredients:

- 4 carrots, peeled and cut into sticks
- 4 cucumbers, peeled and cut into 4 pieces lengthwise
- 3 celery stalks, thinly sliced and lengthwise
- 1 cup of cooked chickpeas
- 3 tablespoons of homemade vegan mayonnaise
- 2 tablespoons of pesto
- 1 teaspoon of cilantro
- a few leaves of thyme
- a few basil leaves
- 1 teaspoon of garlic powder

- 3 tablespoons of rosemary flavored oil
- 1 drizzle of seed oil

Directions:

Put the carrots, cucumbers, and celery in a bowl. Add the flavored oil and mix. With an immersion blender, blend the chickpeas with a drizzle of seed oil; try to get a dense and homogeneous mixture; your humus will be the basis of the other condiments. Pour it over your vegetables, add the pesto and mayonnaise, and mix. Season with coriander, thyme, and basil. If you wish, add the garlic powder and mix. Serve cool.

Nutritional Values: Calories: 77 kcal / Carbohydrates 28g / Protein 6g / Fat 2g / Fiber 38g

Champignon Risotto

Total time: 45 mins / **Prep Time** 10 mins / **Cooking time:** 35 mins / **Difficulty:** Easy

Serving size: 10

Ingredients:

- 3 cups of brown rice
- 2 cups of fresh mushrooms
- 1 ounce of parsley
- 3 ounces of butter
- 1 onion
- 1 tablespoon of chives
- 1 teaspoon of onion powder
- 1 teaspoon of garlic powder
- 1 glass of white wine
- salt and black pepper for seasoning

Directions:

Peel and cut the onion into small slices. Put it in a pan with butter and sauté briefly. As soon as it turns golden, add the mushrooms with parsley and garlic powder. When they start to release their liquids, add the rice and a drizzle of water. Try to keep it boiling by adjusting the flame. Cook for about 25-35 minutes until the rice is well cooked. Stir constantly, and don't let the rice stick to the pan. When you finish cooking, add the chives to the white wine and season with salt and black pepper to taste.

Nutritional Values: Calories: 114 kcal / Carbohydrates 42g / Protein 18g / Fat 13g / Fiber 7g

Roasted Zucchini

Total time: 40 mins / **Prep Time** 10 mins / **Cooking time:** 30 mins / **Difficulty:** Easy

Serving size: 6

Ingredients:

- 8 courgettes
- 2 tablespoons of garlic cream
- 1 teaspoon of red pepper
- 1 lemon, cut in half
- salt and black pepper grains
- Greek yogurt
- salt

Directions:

Cut the courgettes into vertical strips. Preheat your grill or pan where you intend to cook them; in the meantime, spread the garlic cream over each slice and add salt and chili. Cook 15 minutes on each side, and when they start to turn dark, put them in a large bowl. Season with lemon juice or even small pieces and a drizzle of yogurt. Serve hot
Nutritional Values: Calories: 56 kcal / Carbohydrates 38g / Protein 5g / Fat 12g / Fiber 44g

Sweet Pepper Cream

Total time: 45 mins / **Prep Time** 10 mins / **Cooking time:** 35 mins / **Difficulty:** Easy

Serving size: 8

Ingredients:

- 18 slices of 5-grain bread
- 2 yellow peppers
- 3 red peppers
- 4 potatoes, peeled and cut into cubes
- 1 tomato, quartered
- 1 teaspoon of onion powder
- 1 teaspoon of Italian dressing
- salt

Directions:

Put the peppers cut in a saucepan without green stalk and internal seeds. Add the potatoes, tomatoes, salt, and water. Bring to a boil and cook for about 30-35 minutes. Wait for it to thicken and eliminate any moisture. When you finish cooking, add the onion powder and the Italian seasoning. Serve on the plate with the slices of bread.
Nutritional Values: Calories: 77 kcal / Carbohydrates 26g / Protein 11g / Fat 2g / Fiber 36g

Banana Smoothie

Total time: 10 mins / **Prep Time** 10 mins / **Cooking time:** / **Difficulty:** Easy

Serving size: 4

Ingredients:

- 3 bananas
- 3 tablespoons of maple syrup
- 2 tablespoons of cypress honey
- 1 jar of plain yogurt
- a few mint leaves
- 1/2 ounce of strawberries, washed, without small greens, and chopped

Directions:

In a food processor, put the bananas with the strawberries. Add the maple syrup and yogurt. Blend for about twenty seconds. Add honey and serve in a glass with mint. Serve cool
Nutritional Values: Calories: 78 kcal / Carbohydrates 32g / Protein 6g / Fat 1g / Fiber 39g

Banana and Coconut Juice

Total time: 10 mins / **Prep Time** 10 mins / **Cooking time:** / **Difficulty:** Easy

Serving size: 5

Ingredients:

- 3 bananas, peeled and cut into pieces
- 1 coconut, without peel and brown skin
- 2 yellow apples, peeled and seeded, and quartered
- 1 tablespoon of wildflower honey
- 2 lemon slices for serving

- 1/2 cup of almond milk
- 3 tablespoons of blackberries

Directions:

Put the bananas, apples, and coconut in a food processor, add the almond milk and blend for 25 seconds. When finished, filter and collect the juices. For example, you can use the fibrous part for other recipes to make a cake. Put the filtrate in a bowl, add the honey and blackberries and mix. Serve cold with some mint leaves.

Nutritional Values: Calories: 82 kcal / Carbohydrates 18g / Protein 4g / Fat 1g / Fiber 2g

Tomato Cream with Quinoa

Total time: 3 hours / **Prep Time** 30 mins / **Cooking time:** 150 mins / **Difficulty:** Easy

Serving size: 6

Ingredients:

- 3 cups of quinoa
- 1 pound of tomatoes
- 6 potatoes, peeled and thinly sliced
- 2 tablespoons of tomato paste
- 2 carrots, peeled and grated
- 1 onion, thinly sliced
- 1 tablespoon of Italian dressing
- 1 tablespoon of garlic powder
- salt

Directions:

Put the water and salt in a saucepan, bring to a boil and cook the quinoa for about 15 minutes. Next, prepare the tomato cream by putting them in a saucepan with the onion and salt, filling it with water, and bring to a boil. Cook for about 2 hours. Remove the tomato skin and add the potatoes and carrots. Continue cooking for another 40 minutes or so. When finished, mix with the quinoa, add the Italian seasoning and garlic powder, season with salt and serve the creamy quinoa.

Nutritional Values: Calories: 94 kcal / Carbohydrates 38g / Protein 12g / Fat 2g / Fiber 18g

Green Sweet Creamy Zucchini

Total time: 40 mins / **Prep Time** 10 mins / **Cooking time:** 30 mins / **Difficulty:** Easy

Serving size: 8

Ingredients:

- 8 whole meal rolls, rustic
- 4 zucchini, peeled and grated
- 2 potatoes, peeled and thinly sliced
- 1/2 onion
- 1 tablespoon of garlic powder
- 2 tablespoons of chives
- salt

Directions:

In a saucepan, put the zucchini with the potatoes and onion, fill about halfway with water, add the salt and bring to a boil. Cook for about 30 minutes. When done, transfer your salted cream to a blender and blend for a few seconds. There is no need to mix for a long time. Season with garlic powder and chives to taste. Spread the cream on your sandwiches and serve.

Nutritional Values: Calories: 88 kcal / Carbohydrates 36g / Protein 2g / Fat 1g / Fiber 21g

CHAPTER 9: MAIN RECIPES

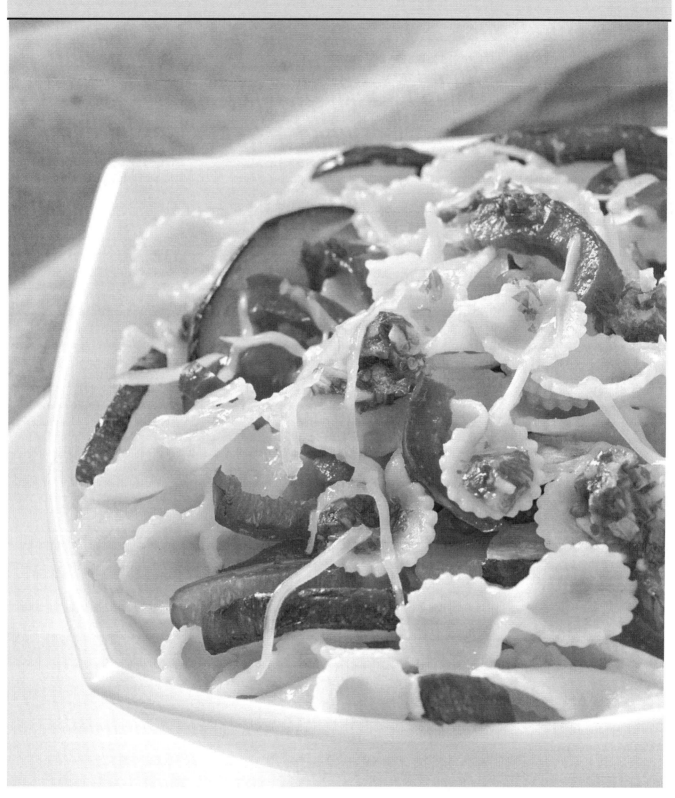

Mashed cauliflower

Total time: 30 mins / **Prep Time** 10 mins /
Cooking time: 20 mins / **Difficulty:** Easy

Serving size: 6

Ingredients:

- 1 drizzle of oil
- 1 head of cauliflower
- 1 potato, peeled
- 1 bunch of red radicchio
- 1/2 cup cooked corn.
- salt

Directions:

Wash the cauliflower and cut the tops. Cook them for 20 minutes in a medium saucepan with the finely chopped potatoes. Then add water and sell. After 20 minutes, remove the water and put the cauliflower and potatoes in a food processor. Blend until you get a thick mixture. In a large bowl, cut the radicchio and mix it with the corn. Add a drizzle of oil and salt and add the cauliflower puree. Serve at room temperature.
Nutritional Values: Calories: 87 kcal / Carbohydrates 18g / Protein 10g / Fat 2g / Fiber 25g

Meat Hash

Total time: 30 mins / **Prep Time** 10 mins /
Cooking time: 20 mins / **Difficulty:** Easy

Serving size: 5

Ingredients:

- meat hash
- 1/4 cup squash, diced
- 1/2 cup bacon, chopped
- 2 eggs
- 3 potatoes, peeled and cut into cubes
- 1 eggplant, peeled and cut into cubes
- 1 teaspoon of garlic powder
- 2 ounces of butter
- 1/2 onion, thinly sliced
- salt

Directions:

Put the pumpkin and bacon in a large pan, add the butter and heat. Begin to flavor the bacon, then add the potatoes, onion, eggplant, and a drizzle of water. Cook with the lid on for about 15 minutes. When the cooking is almost done, break 2 eggs on the sides of the pan and cook them for a few minutes. Serve hot.
Nutritional Values: Calories: 133 kcal / Carbohydrates 21g / Protein 34g / Fat 11g / Fiber 6g

Beans

Total time: 20 mins / **Prep Time** 10 mins /
Cooking time: 10 mins / **Difficulty:** Easy

Serving size: 8

Ingredients:

- 3 pounds of cooked beans
- 1 cup of cooked corn
- 3 carrots, peeled and cut into rings
- 1 onion, peeled and sliced
- 1 ounce of seed oil

Directions:

Make a quick sauté of onion with oil and salt and cook briefly for less than 5 minutes. Put the beans and corn in a bowl. Heat in the microwave for about 90 seconds and mix. Add the cooked onion to the bowl and serve.
Nutritional Values: Calories: 112 kcal / Carbohydrates 28g / Protein 41g / Fat 8g / Fiber 22g

Quinoa and Oatmeal

Total time: 35 mins / **Prep Time** 15 mins /
Cooking time: 15 mins / **Difficulty:** Easy

Serving size: 8

Ingredients:

- 2 cups of quinoa
- 2 and 1/2 cups black grapes
- 4 teaspoons of ginger
- zest of one lemon
- 4 teaspoons vanilla
- salt
- 5 ounces maple syrup

- 3 cups of soy milk
- Water
- almond slivers

Directions:

In a saucepan, mix the water with the quinoa, boil it, and pour in the quinoa. Add the salt and agave syrup. Cook for about 20 minutes, and then add the grapes mixed with grated ginger, vanilla, and lemon zest. Cook for another 10 minutes or so. Serve hot, decorated with almond slivers.

Nutritional Values: Calories: 122 kcal / Carbohydrates 31g / Protein 18g / Fat 11g / Fiber 9g

Scrambled tofu e tomato

Total time: 5 mins / **Prep Time** 5 mins / **Cooking time:** 10 mins / **Difficulty:** Easy

Serving size: 4

Ingredients:

- 8 cherry tomatoes
- 1 cup tofu, cut into cubes
- 2 cups couscous, precooked
- 2 tablespoons curry powder
- 1 teaspoon onion powder
- salt

Directions:

In a saucepan, prepare the couscous by mixing it with water. Bring to a boil and turn off the heat. Let it sit for a few minutes so that it increases in volume. Stir in the curry, salt, and onion powder. Briefly cook the tofu with the tomato cut into quarters in a skillet. Stir in the couscous and serve warm.

Nutritional Values: Calories: 122 kcal / Carbohydrates 31g / Protein 18g / Fat 11g / Fiber 9g

Cheeses and Quinoa

Total time: 25 mins / **Prep Time** 10 mins / **Cooking time:** 15 mins / **Difficulty:** Easy

Serving size: 10

Ingredients:

- 4 cups of quinoa
- 1 tablespoon pepper granules

- 1/4 cup aged cheese
- 3 ounces sweet gorgonzola
- 3 ounces aged parmesan cheese
- 3 ounces string cheese
- Salt

Directions:

Put the water with the quinoa in a saucepan, cook for 15 minutes, and drain. Cut the cheeses into cubes and place them in a bowl. Microwave them for about 30 seconds and then mix them with the quinoa. Season with salt, pepper granules and serve warm.

Nutritional Values: Calories: 177 kcal / Carbohydrates 8g / Protein 29g / Fat 21g / Fiber 12g

Squash Hash

Total time: 45 mins / **Prep Time** 10 mins / **Cooking time:** 35 mins / **Difficulty:** Easy

Serving size: 6

Ingredients:

- 1 pumpkin
- 1 cup pistachios
- 4 ounces of chives
- 3 green apples
- 1 onion
- hot sauce for seasoning

Directions:

Peel and dice the squash. Chop the onion finely and put it in the pan with the squash. Start cooking with a drizzle of water and a lid. Add pistachios and the finely chopped chives and diced apple when it starts to soften. Cook for about 30 minutes. Add the hot sauce and mix everything together when all the ingredients are well cooked. Serve hot.

Nutritional Values: Calories: 136 kcal / Carbohydrates 18g / Protein 11g / Fat 9g / Fiber 21g

Sweet Squid

Total time: 40 mins / **Prep Time** 10 mins / **Cooking time:** 30 mins / **Difficulty:** Easy

Serving size: 8

Ingredients:

- 10 squid, clean and without entrails
- 2 potatoes, cooked and finely chopped, without peel
- 1 red pepper
- 1 avocado, seedless and peeled, finely chopped
- 1 ounce of butter
- salt

Directions:

Set your oven to 390 ° F and line a baking sheet with parchment paper. Put the squid in and cook for about 30 minutes. While they are cooking, prepare your sauce by putting the potato and pepper in a food processor. Add the avocado and butter. Blend until you get a homogeneous mixture. Season with salt. When the squid is ready, put them on a plate and add the sauce. Serve hot.

Nutritional Values: Calories: 114 kcal / Carbohydrates 24g / Protein 41g / Fat 28g / Fiber 11g

Roasted Pepper Cream

Total time: 70 mins / **Prep Time** 20 mins / **Cooking time:** 50 mins / **Difficulty:** Easy

Serving size: 14

Ingredients:

- 2 red peppers
- 3 yellow peppers
- 2 green peppers
- 1 avocado, peeled and seeded
- 3 potatoes, peeled and finely chopped
- 1 tablespoon of flour
- salt
- black pepper for seasoning

Directions:

Wash the peppers thoroughly, remove the green stalk and if you wish, keep some seeds to add to your cream at the end. Prepare your grill; make sure you clean it and it's hot. Slice the peppers and cook them on the grill (or in a pan). Make sure each slice is well cooked and lightly burned. While cooking the peppers in a small pot, cook the potatoes with the avocado and flour. Fill it flush with water and salt and bring it to a boil. Wait for the avocado to melt and the potatoes to become soft. When all the peppers are ready, blend

them in a food processor. Mix the blended peppers with the potatoes in a large bowl and season with the black pepper. Give another smoothie with the food processor and keep it in the fridge for up to 4 days. Alternatively, you can keep it in a sterilized and hermetically sealed jar. Sterilize the pot with your cream and store it in your pantry for 18 months.

Nutritional Values: Calories: 100 kcal / Carbohydrates 29g / Protein 21g / Fat 4g / Fiber 44g

Homemade Mayo

Total time: 10 mins / **Prep Time** 10 mins / **Cooking time:** / **Difficulty:** Easy

Serving size: 20

Ingredients:

- 4 eggs
- 3 cups of corn oil
- 4 tablespoons of vinegar
- a pinch of salt

Directions:

Break the eggs into a bowl. Mix the seed oil with the vinegar and salt in a second bowl. Stir vigorously and combine it with the eggs. Now put your mix in a blender and start pulsing repeatedly. Blend until the mixture is uniform and sufficiently dense. Store in the refrigerator for up to 7 days.

Nutritional Values: Calories: 201 kcal / Carbohydrates 17g / Protein 18g / Fat 39g / Fiber 0g

Octopus with green Sauce

Total time: 50 mins / **Prep Time** 10 mins / **Cooking time:** 40 mins / **Difficulty:** Easy

Serving size: 6

Ingredients:

- 1 large octopus
- 2 boiled potatoes, and without peel
- 1 green pepper
- 1 ounce of chives
- 1 teaspoon of onion powder
- salt

Directions:

Cook your octopus by placing it in a large saucepan

with water and salt. Bring to a boil and cook with the lid on low heat for about 40 minutes. When cooked, drain and put it in a bowl. Meanwhile, prepare your alkaline sauce by blending the peppers with the potato in a food processor. Add the chives and onion powder. Cut the octopus as you wish and add a few basil leaves to decorate your dish.

Nutritional Values: Calories: 89 kcal / Carbohydrates 27g / Protein 38g / Fat 9g / Fiber 14g

Grilled Tofu

Total time: 30 mins / **Prep Time** 10 mins / **Cooking time:** 20 mins / **Difficulty:** Easy

Serving size: 6

Ingredients:

- 1.2 pounds of tofu, cut into slices
- 1 onion, peeled and finely chopped
- 1 ounce of butter
- 1 glass of white wine
- 1/2 ounce of chives
- salt
- black pepper for seasoning

Directions:

In a pan, make a quick sauté with the onion and butter. When it is well browned, add the tofu and stir occasionally. Add the chives and white wine and cook for another 15-20 minutes. Season with salt and black pepper and serve hot.

Nutritional Values: Calories: 99 kcal / Carbohydrates 18g / Protein 24g / Fat 3g / Fiber 9g

Fish Salad

Total time: 30 mins / **Prep Time** 5 mins / **Cooking time:** 20 mins / **Difficulty:** Easy

Serving size: 3

Ingredients:

- 1 raw sea bass, without entrails
- 1 can of tuna
- 2 cups of tomato
- 1/2 cup cooked corn
- 1/4 cup of green lettuce leaves

- a drizzle of oil
- 1/8 cup of vinegar
- salt

Directions:

Cut the fish in half with a knife and put it in a pan. Cook with a bit of water and lid for 20 minutes. When it is ready, let it cool and remove the skin and, with the help of a fork, start scraping the pulp. Be careful to get rid of the thorns. Put the sea bass with the tuna in a bowl, add the tomato cut into 4 parts, and the corn. Add the green lettuce and season with oil, salt, and vinegar drizzle. Serve fresh

Nutritional Values: Calories: 77 kcal / Carbohydrates 15g / Protein 48g / Fat 12g / Fiber 22g

Simple Carpaccio

Total time: 2 hours / **Prep Time** 5 mins / **Cooking time:** / **Difficulty:** Easy

Serving size: 6

Ingredients:

- 12 slices of swordfish, thin
- 1 lemon
- 1 ounce of chives
- 1 tablespoon of parsley leaves, chopped
- 4 tablespoons of olive oil
- 1 teaspoon of garlic powder
- 3 tablespoons of red tomato sauce
- salt

Directions:

Place the slices of your raw fish on a plate. In a small bowl, prepare the sauce for the marinade by squeezing the lemon and grating a small portion of its peel. Next, add the parsley and olive oil. Finally, add the garlic powder and mix. Sprinkle it over the raw fish and let it marinate for at least 2 hours in the refrigerator. When done, add the chives and sauce on top of the fish. Serve cool.

Nutritional Values: Calories: 89 kcal / Carbohydrates 12g / Protein 39g / Fat 22g / Fiber 3g

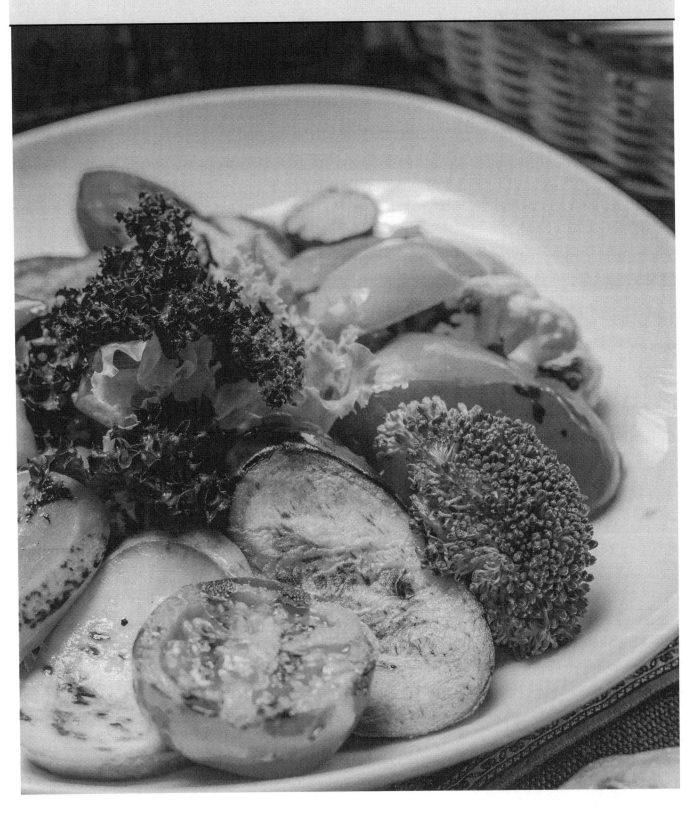

Grilled Vegetables

Total time: 40 mins / **Prep Time** 10 mins / **Cooking time:** 30 mins / **Difficulty:** Easy

Serving size: 5

Ingredients:

- 1 yellow pepper, without stalk and seeds, cut into slices
- 1 onion, cut into 8 parts
- 1/4 pumpkin, sliced
- 1 large aubergine, peeled and sliced
- 1 lemon
- a few leaves of parsley
- 3 tablespoons of raw oil
- salt

Directions:

Start heating your grill; make sure it is clean and there are no residues. Prepare the dressing for the vegetables by placing the lemon juice with parsley and oil in a bowl. Add the salt and mix. Start cooking your vegetables on the grill now; make sure they are well cooked. When ready, place them on a plate and sprinkle the prepared dressing. you serve

Nutritional Values: Calories: 91 kcal / Carbohydrates 29g / Protein 18g / Fat 2g / Fiber 39g

Coconut and mango

Total time: 20 mins / **Prep Time** 20 mins / **Cooking time:** / **Difficulty:** Easy

Serving size: 4

Ingredients:

- 1 large coconut, peeled and without brown skin
- 2 mangoes, peeled and seeded
- 1 head of green cabbage,
- a few fennel leaves
- parsley
- 1 ounce of oil
- 2 leaves of chives

- salt and black pepper for seasoning of raw oil
- salt

Directions:

In a food processor, blend the cabbage with the radicchio, and add the chopped parsley and chives for seasoning. Prepare the coconut with the mango in a bowl, chop them coarsely, add the blended vegetables, and season with the oil. Season with salt and black pepper and serve chilled.

Nutritional Values: Calories: 88 kcal / Carbohydrates 34g / Protein 22g / Fat 6g / Fiber 40g

Simple Basil Quinoa

Total time: 20 mins / **Prep Time** 5 mins / **Cooking time:** 15 mins / **Difficulty:** Easy

Serving size: 6

Ingredients:

- 3 cups of quinoa
- 1/2 cup of basil
- 2 ounces of oil
- 1/2 cup soft cheese, grated
- black pepper for seasoning
- salt

Directions:

Put the water and salt in a saucepan and bring to a boil. Cook the quinoa for about 15 minutes. Drain and put in a bowl. While the quinoa is cooking, finely chop the washed basil and mix it with the cheese and pepper. Drizzle with oil and mix. When the quinoa is ready, add the prepared dressing and mix. Serve hot blended vegetables, and season with the oil. Season with salt and black pepper and serve chilled.

Nutritional Values: Calories: 94 kcal / Carbohydrates 28g / Protein 28g / Fat 8g / Fiber 34g

Vegetable Toast

Total time: 15 mins / **Prep Time** 5 mins / **Cooking time:** 10 mins / **Difficulty:** Easy

Serving size: 4

Ingredients:

- 8 slices of toast bread

- 1/4 cup of salsa Verde
- 1/3 head of green cabbage, chopped
- 1 teaspoon of chives
- 1 eggplant, peeled, thinly sliced, and cooked
- 2 grated carrots

Directions:

Using a knife, spread the green sauce on 4 slices, add the cabbage, a few pieces of eggplant, and the chives, and finish with the grated carrots. Close with a second slice and cook for about 10 minutes. Serve hot
Nutritional Values: Calories: 98 kcal / Carbohydrates 34g / Protein 14g / Fat 6g / Fiber 32g

Homemade Bread

Total time: 3 hours / **Prep Time** 20 mins / **Cooking time:** 50 mins / **Difficulty:** Easy

Serving size: 8

Ingredients:

- 4 cups of whole meal flour
- 1 cube of yeast for bread
- salt
- 1 ounce of olive oil
- 1/2 cup black olives, pitted

Directions:

Put the flour with the salt in a bowl and add the yeast. Gently start adding the water and knead with your hands. Next, add the black olives and oil. The total amount of water usually is just under half. If the dough is too liquid, add a few more tablespoons of flour; otherwise, keep it and let it rise. It usually takes 60-120 minutes for a complete leavening. When it has risen well, turn the oven to 395 ° F and bake your loaves of bread for about 45-50 minutes. When finished, let it rest in a tea towel and store it in a dry place.
Nutritional Values: Calories: 104 kcal / Carbohydrates 41g / Protein 21g / Fat 3g / Fiber 26g

Green anti-inflammatory roasted salad

Total time: 40 mins / **Prep Time** 5 mins / **Cooking time:** 35 mins / **Difficulty:** Easy

Serving size: 6

Ingredients:

- 10 courgettes, washed and cut lengthwise
- 1 head of white cabbage
- 2 carrots
- 1 stalk of celery
- 1 tablespoon of garlic powder
- 1 tablespoon of onion powder
- salt
- black pepper
- chopped parsley
- 1 ounce of oil
- juice of 1 lemon

Directions:

In a food processor, blend the tops of the white cabbage, add the carrots and celery and continue to blend. Season the blended vegetables with garlic and onion powder and black pepper. Now heat your grill and arrange the courgettes on top when hot. Cook for 15-20 minutes on each side. When well cooked, place on the plate and mix with the seasoning. Finally, prepare the lemon sauce by mixing the oil with the parsley and lemon in a bowl. Sprinkle over the entire plate with a silicone brush. Enjoy your meal.
Nutritional Values: Calories: 80 kcal / Carbohydrates 37g / Protein 13g / Fat 7g / Fiber 38g

Fresh Spelled Avocado Salad

Total time: 30 mins / **Prep Time** 10 mins / **Cooking time:** 20 mins / **Difficulty:** Easy

Serving size: 4

Ingredients:

- 2 cups of spelled
- 4 tomatoes, cut into 4
- 1/2 cup of corn
- 2 avocados, peeled and seeded
- 1/2 onion, finely chopped
- salt

- black pepper for seasoning

- 1/3 of your favorite sweet and sour sauce

Directions:

In a saucepan, put the water with the salt and bring it to a boil. Pour the spelled with the onion and cook for about 15-20 minutes. Prepare your dressing by placing diced avocado with corn in a bowl. Add the sweet and sour sauce of your choice and the tomato. When the spell is ready, drain it and add it to the sauce. Season with salt and black pepper and serve cold.

Nutritional Values: Calories: 84 kcal / Carbohydrates 42g / Protein 18g / Fat 5g / Fiber 39g

Vegan spring roll

Total time: 55 mins / **Prep Time** 20 mins / **Cooking time:** 35 mins / **Difficulty:** Easy

Serving size: 8

Ingredients:

- 1 cup of flour

- 1 tablespoon of cornstarch

- salt

- 1 head of green cabbage

- 3 carrots, peeled

- 3 tablespoons of bean sprouts

- 1 teaspoon of onion powder

- 1 courgette, peeled and pulped

- some radicchio leaves

Directions:

Prepare the dough for your rolls by mixing the flour with the cornstarch and salt in a bowl. Gently add the water and start kneading with your hands. The mixture must be homogeneous and must not be sticky. Prepare the seasonings by putting the cabbage florets in a blender and add the carrots and courgette pulp. Blend repeatedly for a few seconds. Roll out your dough over a large surface and add the prepared toppings. Season with the onion powder and bean sprouts, and finish with a red radicchio leaf. Roll the rolls to one side. Preheat the oven to 380 ° F and line a baking sheet with parchment paper. Transfer the registrations to the baking sheet and bake for 30-35 minutes or until the dough is golden brown. Serve hot.

Nutritional Values: Calories: 112 kcal /

Carbohydrates 36g / Protein 8g / Fat 2g / Fiber 37g

Vegetables Spring

Total time: 20 mins / **Prep Time** 20 mins / **Cooking time:** / **Difficulty:** Easy

Serving size: 3

Ingredients:

- 1/2 head of green cabbage

- 1/4 cup of green lettuce

- 1/2 cup of corn

- 1 stalk of chopped celery

- 1/2 head of red radicchio

- Salted yogurt, natural

- 3 tablespoons of raw oil

- salt (to taste)

Directions:

Wash all your vegetables, blend the kale and arrange the lettuce leaves on the plate. Put the mixed cabbage in with the corn and chopped celery. With a knife, cut the radicchio leaves and add them to the dish. Season with the yogurt and oil and add salt if you wish. Serve cool.

Nutritional Values: Calories: 79 kcal / Carbohydrates 34g / Protein 6g / Fat 9g / Fiber 44

Boiled Potato

Total time: 30 mins / **Prep Time** 10 mins / **Cooking time:** 20 mins / **Difficulty:** Easy

Serving size: 8

Ingredients:

- 4 cups of potatoes, peeled and cut into cubes

- 1/8 cup of parsley leaves

- Salt

- Black pepper granules

Directions:

In a large saucepan, place potatoes with water. Add salt and bring to a boil. Cook for about 18 to 20 minutes, until potatoes flake slightly. Drain and stir in parsley and black pepper. Serve hot or cold as a side dish with green vegetables.

Nutritional Values: Calories: 92 kcal / Carbohydrates 18g / Protein 7g / Fat 1g / Fiber 15g

Roasted Onion

Total time: 30 mins / **Prep Time** 5 mins / **Cooking time:** 25 mins / **Difficulty:** Easy

Serving size: 4

Ingredients:

- 6 medium onions, peeled and cut into 8 pieces
- a few leaves of parsley
- 1 ounce of oil
- juice of 1 lemon
- 1 teaspoon of hot pepper
- salt

Directions:

Prepare your grill and arrange the onions on top when it is hot. Cook on each side for about 20-25 minutes or until cooked. While the onions are cooking, prepare the dressing by putting the lemon juice with the oil and parsley in a small bowl. Add the hot pepper and stir for a few seconds. Place the onions in a dish and sprinkle the prepared dressing. Serve hot

Nutritional Values: Calories: 84 kcal / Carbohydrates 12g / Protein 2g / Fat 0g / Fiber 29g

Spinach with Garlic

Total time: 30 mins / **Prep Time** 10 mins / **Cooking time:** 20 mins / **Difficulty:** Easy

Serving size: 6

Ingredients:

- 1 large packet of frozen spinach
- 8-10 cloves of garlic
- 1 ounce of butter
- 1 teaspoon of onion powder
- 1 teaspoon of garlic powder
- 1 tablespoon of Italian dressing
- salt and black pepper for seas

Directions:

In a pan, make a quick sauté with the garlic and butter. When the garlic starts to brown, add the spinach and a drizzle of water, and cook with the lid on for about 20 minutes. Wait until the spinach is cooked through. Halfway through cooking, add the onion and garlic powder and finish with the Italian dressing. After 20 minutes, remove the lid and wait until all the liquids have almost evaporated. Complete your dish by adding salt and black pepper to taste. Serve hot.

Nutritional Values: Calories: 97 kcal / Carbohydrates 18g / Protein 18g / Fat 4g / Fiber 32g

Coconut and Avocado

Total time: 10 mins / **Prep Time** 10 mins / **Cooking time:** / **Difficulty:** Easy

Serving size: 5

Ingredients:

- 1 coconut, peeled and skinless brown, sliced
- 2 avocados, without skin and seeds and cut into 4 parts
- 2 tablespoons of honey
- 1/2 cup of whole grains
- 3 tablespoons of agave syrup

Directions:

Place the avocado cut into about 1.5-inch pieces in a bowl. Blend the coconut and mix it with the avocado. Add honey and whole grains and mix. Finally, mix with the agave syrup and serve fresh.

Nutritional Values: Calories: 124 kcal / Carbohydrates 38g / Protein 16g / Fat 9g / Fiber 39g

Healthy Anti-inflammatory Salad

Total time: 20 mins / **Prep Time** 20 mins / **Cooking time:** / **Difficulty:** Easy

Serving size: 4

Ingredients:

- 1 head of green cabbage
- 5 tomatoes, quartered
- 2 red apples, cut into 8 parts with the peel
- 1 teaspoon of Italian dressing
- 1 hard green pear, cut into 8 parts with the peel
- 1 drizzle of coconut oil
- 2 tablespoons of chopped walnuts

- 2 tablespoons of toasted almonds
- salt

Directions:

In a large bowl, put the cabbage and tomatoes. Add the sliced apples and pears and drizzle with the coconut oil and Italian dressing. Stir and finally add the dried fruit. Season with salt and serve cool

Nutritional Values: Calories: 90 kcal / Carbohydrates 22g / Protein 16g / Fat 3g / Fiber 30g

Sweet Beetroot

Total time: 15 mins / **Prep Time** 15 mins / **Cooking time:** / **Difficulty:** Easy

Serving size: 7

Ingredients:

- sweet beetroot
- 2 beets, cooked and peeled
- 2 ounces of chives
- 2 tablespoons of raw corn oil
- 1 ounce of flax seeds, finely chopped
- 2 carrots, peeled and cut into ring

Directions:

In a bowl, put the beetroot cut into cubes. Add the carrot and season with the oil and chives. Finish by placing the flax seeds. Serve fresh.

Nutritional Values: Calories: 68 kcal / Carbohydrates 19g / Protein 17g / Fat 3g / Fiber 34g

CHAPTER 11: SALAD RECIPES

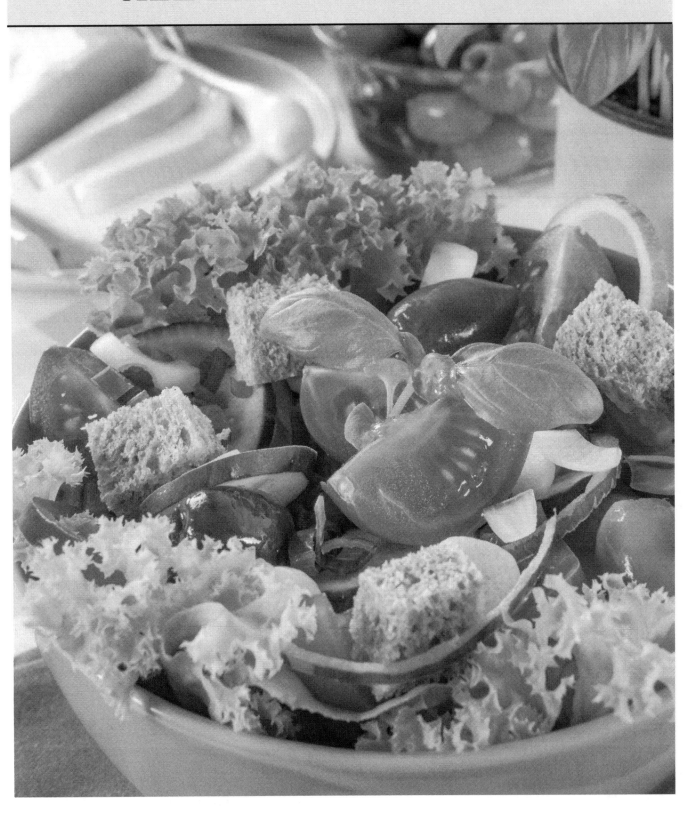

Green Simple Salad

Total time: 10 mins / **Prep Time** 10 mins / **Cooking time:** / **Difficulty:** Easy

Serving size: 5

Ingredients:

- 1 large bunch of green lettuce
- 1/2 bunch of white cabbage
- 1/2 bunch of cooked cauliflower
- 2 carrots, peeled and cut into rings
- 2 tablespoons of sweet soy sauce
- 1/2 glass (1 ounce) of white wine vinegar
- 2 tablespoons of bean sprouts
- salt

Directions:

In a large salad bowl, cut the lettuce leaves. Blend the white cabbage and add the cauliflower florets. Add the carrots and mix. Before serving, season with the soy sauce, vinegar, and, if desired, the bean sprouts. Top with salt and serve chilled.

Nutritional Values: Calories: 88 kcal / Carbohydrates 35g / Protein 12g / Fat 3g / Fiber 41g

Tofu vegan Salad

Total time: 20 mins / **Prep Time** 10 mins / **Cooking time:** 10 mins / **Difficulty:** Easy

Serving size: 7

Ingredients:

- 1 large packet of tofu, plain
- 1/2 onion, finely chopped
- 1 tablespoon of seed oil
- 1 red pepper
- 1 green pepper
- 1/2 head of cabbage, pureed
- 1 teaspoon of garlic powder
- 1 teaspoon of Italian dressing
- salt

Directions:

Make a quick sauté with the onion and oil in a pan, and season with the garlic powder, the Italian seasoning, and salt if desired. When well browned, add the tofu and lower the heat. If necessary, also add a little water. Stir occasionally. In a salad bowl, finely chop the peppers, remove the seeds and add the cabbage. Stir and finally add the tofu. Serve

Nutritional Values: Calories: 95 kcal / Carbohydrates 34g / Protein 18g / Fat 6g / Fiber 39g

Seitan Salad

Total time: 15 mins / **Prep Time** 10 mins / **Cooking time:** 5 mins / **Difficulty:** Easy

Serving size: 4

Ingredients:

- 1/2 bunch of green lettuce
- 1 small bunch of red radicchio
- 1/4 cup of blackberries
- 1 packet of seitan, 4 slices in total
- 2 tablespoons of white sauce, sweet
- 1 teaspoon of Italian dressing
- salt

Directions:

In a pan, briefly heat the seitan (about 5 minutes). While it is heating up, prepare the salad by mixing the lettuce and radicchio in a salad bowl. Add the blackberries and drizzle with the white sauce. When ready, put the seitan on a plate and add a generous portion of vegetables. Season with salt to taste.

Nutritional Values: Calories: 98 kcal / Carbohydrates 32g / Protein 26g / Fat 3g / Fiber 38g

Potatoes Salad

Total time: 25 mins / **Prep Time** 10 mins / **Cooking time:** 15 mins / **Difficulty:** Easy

Serving size: 8

Ingredients:

- 2 pounds of potatoes, peeled
- a few leaves of parsley, chopped
- 1 teaspoon of garlic powder
- 1/2 cup of white wine vinegar
- 2 teaspoons of black pepper

- salt

Directions:

Cut the potatoes into large cubes. Put the water with the salt in a saucepan and bring it to a boil. Add the potatoes and cook for 10-15 minutes; the potatoes should not fall apart. When ready, drain and put them in a large bowl; add the garlic powder and vinegar. Before serving, add the fresh parsley to taste and the black pepper.
Nutritional Values: Calories: 103 kcal / Carbohydrates 40g / Protein 2g / Fat 2g / Fiber 14g

Radicchio Salad

Total time: 25 mins / **Prep Time** 10 mins / **Cooking time:** / **Difficulty:** Easy

Serving size: 10

Ingredients:

- 2 large bunches of red radicchio
- 1 cup of blackberries
- 1/2 cup of red berries
- 1 red pepper
- 3 large tomatoes, quartered
- salt
- raw oil

Directions:

In a large salad bowl, cut the radicchio leaves as you like, add the black and red berries and mix. Next, cut the pepper into small strips, remove the seeds and add them to the tomato salad. Before serving, season with oil and salt.
Nutritional Values: Calories: 50 kcal / Carbohydrates 18g / Protein 4g / Fat 1g / Fiber 34g

Tomatoes Salad

Total time: 10 mins / **Prep Time** 10 mins / **Cooking time:** / **Difficulty:** Easy

Serving size: 12

Ingredients:

- 8 large tomatoes, cut into 4
- 2 tablespoons of capers
- 1 stick of rosemary, only the leaves

- 1 teaspoon of Italian dressing
- 1 tablespoon of black pepper granules
- 2 tablespoons of raw oil
- salt

Directions:

In a large bowl, place the tomatoes and season with the Italian dressing. Add the rosemary and capers and the pepper in granules. Before serving, add the salt and the Italian seasoning.
Nutritional Values: Calories: 52 kcal / Carbohydrates 22g / Protein 6g / Fat 2g / Fiber 32g

Champignon Salad

Total time: 30 mins / **Prep Time** 10 mins / **Cooking time:** 20 mins / **Difficulty:** Easy

Serving size: 5

Ingredients:

- 2 cups of champignon mushrooms, washed and sliced
- a few leaves of parsley
- 3 cloves of garlic
- salt
- 1/2 green cabbage, pureed
- 1 teaspoon of black pepper
- 1 teaspoon of Italian dressing
- 1 ounce of seed oil
- salt

Directions:

In a pan, make a quick sauté with oil and crushed garlic. When it starts to brown slightly, add the mushrooms and parsley. Cook over low heat and cover for about 20 minutes, stirring occasionally. When ready, remove the garlic and place the mushrooms in a bowl with paper towels. While the mushrooms are cooking, blend the green cabbage and season with the black pepper and the Italian seasoning. Finally, mix it with the mushrooms and serve. Season with salt to taste.
Nutritional Values: Calories: 77 kcal / Carbohydrates 24g / Protein 12g / Fat 5g / Fiber 18g

Pumpkin Salad

Total time: 35 mins / **Prep Time** 10 mins / **Cooking time:** 25 mins / **Difficulty:** Easy

Serving size: 8

Ingredients:

- 1 giant pumpkin, sliced and seeded
- 2 ounces of butter
- 1 tablespoon of seed oil
- 1 tablespoon of garlic powder
- 1 tablespoon of Italian dressing
- 1 green onion, thinly sliced
- salt and black pepper for seasoning

Directions:

In a large saucepan, sauté the onion and butter quickly. When it starts to brown, put the pumpkin slices in and cook with a lid for about 20-25 minutes. Halfway through cooking, add the garlic powder and the Italian seasoning. When the pumpkin is well cooked, put it in a bowl, add the oil, and season with salt and black pepper to taste. Serve warm or even excellent.

Nutritional Values: Calories: 88 kcal / Carbohydrates 32g / Protein 16g / Fat 3g / Fiber 22g

Zucchini Salad

Total time: 25 mins / **Prep Time** 10 mins / **Cooking time:** 15 mins / **Difficulty:** Easy

Serving size: 3

Ingredients:

- 4 courgettes, cut into rings
- 1 bunch of green lettuce
- 1 red pepper, thinly sliced and seedless
- 1 teaspoon of Italian dressing
- 1/2 onion, finely chopped

Directions:

In a pan, cook the courgettes and onion for 10-15 minutes, with a drizzle of water and the lid on. Next, prepare the salad with the pepper and the lettuce cut as you wish. Add the Italian dressing. When the courgettes are ready, pour them into the salad and mix everything. Season to taste. Serve.

Nutritional Values: Calories: 55 kcal / Carbohydrates 28g / Protein 12g / Fat 6g / Fiber 29g

Boiled Endive Salad

Total time: 25 mins / **Prep Time** 5 mins / **Cooking time:** 20 mins / **Difficulty:** Easy

Serving size: 6

Ingredients:

- 1 large bunch of endive (about 1.5 lbs.)
- 2 tablespoons of olive oil
- salt
- black pepper for seasoning

Directions:

In a saucepan, put the water with the salt and bring it to a boil. When it boils, add the vegetables and lower the heat. Cook for about 20 minutes, stirring occasionally. When finished, remove the water and place the vegetables in a large bowl. Season with oil and black pepper, and season with salt before serving.

Nutritional Values: Calories: 40 kcal / Carbohydrates 10g / Protein 2g / Fat 0g / Fiber 38g

Organic Meat Salad

Total time: 40 mins / **Prep Time** 15 mins / **Cooking time:** 25 mins / **Difficulty:** Easy

Serving size: 5

Ingredients:

- 5 slices of organic meat
- 1 bunch of green lettuce
- 1 lemon
- chopped parsley
- 2 tablespoons of oil

Directions:

Cook the meat in a pan for 20-25 minutes with water and a lid. The heart must be boiled and not roasted. When tender, place it in a bowl and cut it into about 1-inch pieces. While the meat is cooking, prepare the sauce by putting the parsley, lemon juice, and oil in a bowl. Mix and pour over the meat when ready. Serve on the plate with the lettuce.

Nutritional Values: Calories: 88 kcal / Carbohydrates 6g / Protein 28g / Fat 3g / Fiber 2g

Green Bean Salad

Total time: 45 mins / **Prep Time** 30 mins / **Cooking time:** 15 mins / **Difficulty:** Easy

Serving size: 8

Ingredients:

- 2 pounds of green beans
- 4 tomatoes, cut into 4 parts
- 1 tablespoon of capers in oil
- 4 artichoke hearts in oil
- salt and black pepper for seasoning
- 4 boiled eggs cut into 2 or 4 parts
- salt

Directions:

Remove the tips of the green beans with the help of scissors. In a saucepan, bring the water with salt to a boil. Add the green beans and cook for about 15 minutes as soon as it boils. Drain the water and place them in the bowl when they are tender. Add the cherry tomatoes and season with the capers and artichokes. Add the boiled eggs and season with salt and black pepper. Serve also at room temperature.
Nutritional Values: Calories: 77 kcal / Carbohydrates 18g / Protein 12g / Fat 0g / Fiber 36g

Yellow Salad

Total time: 30 mins / **Prep Time** 30 mins / **Cooking time:** / **Difficulty:** Easy

Serving size: 5

Ingredients:

- 2 yellow peppers
- 1 cup of sweetcorn, cooked
- 1 yellow apple, washed and thinly sliced
- 1 lemon

- 3 tablespoons of bean sprouts
- salt

Directions:

In a large salad bowl, place the finely chopped, seedless peppers. Add the corn and apple slices. Squeeze the lemon to dress your salad and grate over the peel if you wish. Add the bean sprouts, and before serving, add the salt.
Nutritional Values: Calories: 88 kcal / Carbohydrates 32g / Protein 18g / Fat 2g / Fiber 44g

Legumes Mix Salad

Total time: 10 mins / **Prep Time** 10 mins / **Cooking time:** / **Difficulty:** Easy

Serving size: 6

Ingredients:

- 1/2 cup of cooked beans
- 1/2 cup cooked lentils
- 1/2 cup of cooked chickpeas
- 1 bunch of red radicchio
- 1 bunch of green lettuce
- 2 red peppers
- 1 ounce of raw oil
- 1 tablespoon of Italian dressing
- salt

Directions:

In a large bowl, put all the legumes. Make sure you get the liquids out of the jar. Cut the lettuce leaves to the size you want and add the sliced, seedless red peppers. Season with oil and Italian seasoning, and finally, season with salt.
Nutritional Values: Calories: 99 kcal / Carbohydrates 13g / Protein 42g / Fat 3g / Fiber 36g

CHAPTER 12: POULTRY RECIPES

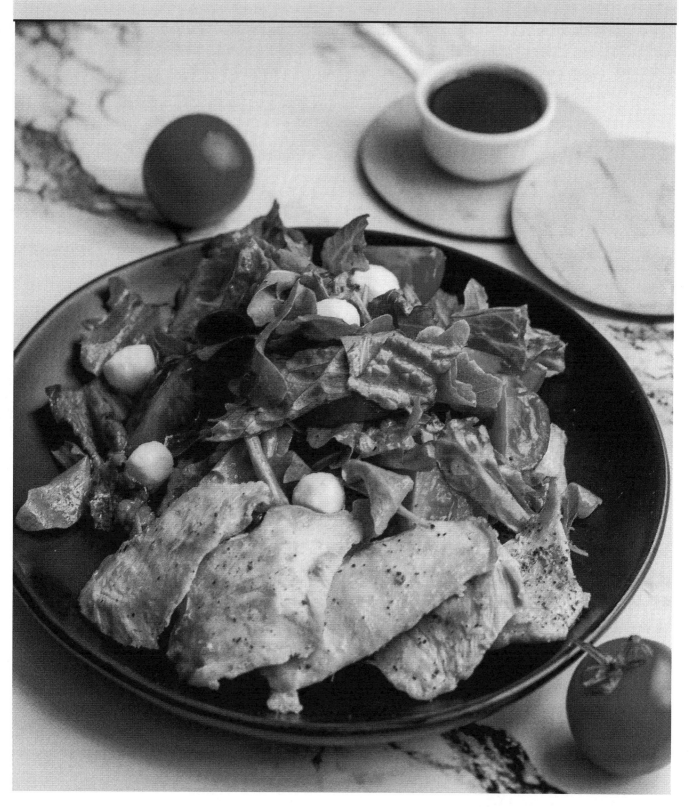

Breaded Chicken

Total time: 30 mins / **Prep Time** 10 mins /
Cooking time: 20 mins / **Difficulty:** Easy

Serving size: 3

Ingredients:

- 3 slices of chicken breast
- 1 egg
- 1/4 cup of breadcrumbs
- 1 teaspoon of garlic powder
- 1 teaspoon of Italian dressing
- a few chopped parsley leaves
- salt
- black pepper
- Fry oil

Directions:

In a small bowl, beat the egg and mix for a few seconds, adding a pinch of salt. In a dish, prepare the crumb by mixing it with the garlic powder and the Italian dressing. Add a few leaves of parsley, salt, and pepper. Mix. Dip the chicken slices first in the egg and then in the seasoned crumb. Heat the oil in a skillet and cook the chicken on both sides. Serve hot.
You can also cook the breaded chicken in the air fryer for 10-15 minutes per side at 390 ° F. Serve.
Nutritional Values: Calories: 115 kcal / Carbohydrates 6g / Protein 29g / Fat 4g / Fiber 2g

Chicken with green Sauce

Total time: 20 mins / **Prep Time** 10 mins /
Cooking time: 10 mins / **Difficulty:** Easy

Serving size: 6

Ingredients:

- 6 slices of boneless chicken
- 1 avocado
- a few leaves of parsley
- 1 boiled potato and without peel
- 1 green pepper
- 1 tablespoon of salted butter
- 1 tablespoon of seed oil

- 2 tablespoons of basil leaves

Directions:

In a pan, cook the chicken slices with a drizzle of water and a lid. Cook for 10 minutes over medium heat. While the chicken is cooking, make your own sauce. Put the sliced, seeded pepper in a blender. Add the avocado and potato. Blend and add the butter with oil and basil. Blend until you get a homogeneous mixture. When the chicken is ready, place it on a plate and serve with the freshly prepared sauce.
Nutritional Values: Calories: 120 kcal / Carbohydrates 4g / Protein 32g / Fat 9g / Fiber 8g

Grilled Chicken

Total time: 45 mins / **Prep Time** 10 mins /
Cooking time: 35 mins / **Difficulty:** Easy

Serving size: 7

Ingredients:

- 7 slices of chicken, boneless
- 1 lemon
- 1/2 cup of vinegar
- 1 ounce of chives
- 1/4 cup of oil
- salt

Directions:

Prepare your grill and put the chicken on top when it's hot. Cook for about 15-20 minutes on each side. Grid each part well. While the chicken is cooking, prepare the dressing by mixing the vinegar with the oil and chives in a bowl. Add a pinch of salt. When the chicken is well cooked, place it on a plate and brush over the prepared sauce. Serve hot
Nutritional Values: Calories: 110 kcal / Carbohydrates 6g / Protein 34g / Fat 13g / Fiber 4g

Spicy Chicken

Total time: 25 mins / **Prep Time** 10 mins /
Cooking time: 15 mins / **Difficulty:** Easy

Serving size: 5

Ingredients:

- 1 large, boneless chicken
- 3 finely chopped tomatoes
- 3 cloves of garlic, crushed

- 1 teaspoon of red pepper
- 1 ounce of chives
- a few leaves of parsley, chopped
- 1 tablespoon of gelatin
- 1 ounce of oil

Directions:

Put the chicken in a saucepan and add a drizzle of water. Cook with the lid on for 10-15 minutes; the meat should turn white. While it cooks, make your own spicy sauce. In a small bowl, put the chives and mix them with the parsley and oil. In a mortar (or food processor), blend the tomato with the garlic and add it to the sauce bowl. Add the gelatin and mix for a few minutes. When the chicken is cooked, turn off the heat and put the sauce into the pot. Let it rest for a few minutes and serve hot.

Nutritional Values: Calories: 132 kcal / Carbohydrates 12g / Protein 37g / Fat 13g / Fiber 4g

Stuffed Chicken

Total time: 25 mins / **Prep Time** 10 mins / **Cooking time:** 50 mins / **Difficulty:** Medium

Serving size: 8

Ingredients:

- 1 large boneless chicken
- 1 pound of potatoes, peeled and cut into small slices or cubes

For the dressing:

- 1 bell pepper
- 1/2 head of cabbage
- 1 head of green broccoli
- 3 carrots, peeled

Directions:

Prepare the dressing by peeling the pepper and removing its seeds. Blend the cabbage first, the broccoli, and the carrots with the pepper. Put all the ingredients in a bowl and mix quickly. Put the components inside the chicken using your hands and close with a food string. Set the oven to 400 ° F and prepare your baking sheet with cart for no. Put the potatoes and the chicken with the filling on top. Cook for about 50 minutes or until the chicken is well cooked and its meat tender. Serve hot.

Nutritional Values: Calories: 150 kcal /

Carbohydrates 11g / Protein 41g / Fat 11g / Fiber 18g

Chicken with Pink Sauce

Total time: 45 mins / **Prep Time** 15 mins / **Cooking time:** 30 mins / **Difficulty:** Easy

Serving size: 3

Ingredients:

- 3 slices of chicken breast
- 4 large tomatoes, sliced
- 2 cloves of garlic, crushed
- 2 teaspoons of onion powder
- 1 teaspoon of Italian dressing
- 2 ounces of soft cheese cubes
- 1/4 cup of Greek yogurt, salted
- 1 potato, boiled
- salt

Directions:

Put the chicken to cook in your pan. Cook for 7-10 minutes on each side. While the chicken is cooking, prepare your sauce by blending the tomatoes with the cheese and finally adding the garlic and onion and the Italian dressing. Mash the potato with a fork and add the Greek yogurt. Adjust with salt. When the chicken is ready, place each slice on a plate and sprinkle the pink sauce on top. Enjoy your meal.

Nutritional Values: Calories: 133 kcal / Carbohydrates 9g / Protein 39g / Fat 14g / Fiber 7g

Cheese Chicken

Total time: 25 mins / **Prep Time** 5 mins / **Cooking time:** 20 mins / **Difficulty:** Easy

Serving size: 7

Ingredients:

- 7 slices of chicken breasts
- 1/2 cup of gorgonzola cheese
- 1/2 cup of soft cheese
- 3 ounces of grated Parmesan cheese
- 1 mozzarella, without liquids
- parsley, a few leaves

Directions:

In a bowl, prepare your cheeses, cutting the soft ones and mozzarella into cubes. Add the parmesan and gorgonzola cut into strips. Now cook the chicken in a pan for 10 minutes per side, and while cooking, put the cheeses prepared previously. Serve hot

Nutritional Values: Calories: 175 kcal / Carbohydrates 11g / Protein 44g / Fat 23g / Fiber 6g

Italian Chicken

Total time: 35 mins / **Prep Time** 5 mins / **Cooking time:** 30 mins / **Difficulty:** Easy

Serving size: 2

Ingredients:

- 2 slices of chicken
- 1/4 cup of breadcrumbs
- 1 egg
- salt and black pepper
- 1 teaspoon of chives
- 3 tablespoons of red tomato sauce

Directions:

In a small bowl, beat the egg. Put the breadcrumbs on a plate and season with the chives, salt, and black pepper. Dip the chicken slices first in the egg and then in the seasoned crumb. Cook in a pan for 15 minutes on each side, and when the chicken is well browned, place it on the plate. Serve it with the fresh sauce on top.

Nutritional Values: Calories: 99 kcal / Carbohydrates 4g / Protein 38g / Fat 11g / Fiber 4g

Chicken Soup

Total time: 80 mins / **Prep Time** 20 mins / **Cooking time:** 60 mins / **Difficulty:** Easy

Serving size: 6

Ingredients:

- 1 large boneless whole chicken
- 1 cup of mushrooms
- 1 stalk of celery
- 1 tablespoon of tomato paste
- 1 cube of meat
- 2 ounces of chives

- 1 teaspoon of garlic powder
- 1 tablespoon of Italian dressing
- oil
- salt

Directions:

Chop the chicken into large chunks and place in a large saucepan. Add the chives and a drizzle of oil. Start cooking by adding the garlic powder as well. After a few minutes, fill the saucepan about 3/4 of the way and bring it to a boil. Turn the flame down and put the lid on. Leave it to a slight bump. Add the mushrooms, celery, and nut and continue cooking. Stir occasionally. Add the Italian condiment to the cooking end and finally season with salt. Serve hot.

Nutritional Values: Calories: 115 kcal / Carbohydrates 12g / Protein 32g / Fat 14g / Fiber 5g

Green Chicken

Total time: 50 mins / **Prep Time** 10 mins / **Cooking time:** 40 mins / **Difficulty:** Easy

Serving size: 8

Ingredients:

- 1 large chicken, boneless
- 1 bunch of broccoli
- 1 head of green cabbage
- 4 carrots, peeled and cut into rings
- 1/2 cup of white wine vinegar
- 1 tablespoon of garlic powder
- 1 tablespoon of onion powder
- Oil
- salt

Directions:

In a saucepan, put the water with the salt and bring it to a boil. Add the chicken and let it cook over low heat for about 40 minutes. As it cooks, prepare the dressing by placing the broccoli and cabbage in a blender. Blend and transfer everything to a bowl. Add the carrots and a drizzle of oil. When the chicken is almost ready, add the vinegar, garlic, and onion powder, season with salt, and when ready, put it in the large bowl with the vegetables. Stir and serve hot.

Nutritional Values: Calories: 124 kcal / Carbohydrates 6g / Protein 38g / Fat 12g / Fiber 14g

Chicken BBQ

Total time: 50 mins / **Prep Time** 10 mins / **Cooking time:** 40 mins / **Difficulty:** Easy

Serving size: 7

Ingredients:

- 1 large, roughly chopped, boneless chicken
- 1/2 cup of soy sauce
- 5 tomatoes
- 3 cloves of garlic
- 1 onion, cut into 4 parts
- 1 teaspoon of Italian dressing
- salt

Directions:

First, prepare your dressing. In a food processor, put the tomatoes with the onion and garlic. Blend and add the Italian dressing. Add a pinch of salt. Next, prepare your BBQ and make sure the grills are clean. Place your chicken and cook for at least 35-40 minutes evenly. When the chicken is ready, spread the seasoning and soy sauce over it to taste. Serve hot.

Nutritional Values: Calories: 117 kcal / Carbohydrates 14g / Protein 39g / Fat 9g / Fiber 8g

Almond Chicken

Total time: 50 mins / **Prep Time** 20 mins / **Cooking time:** 30 mins / **Difficulty:** Easy

Serving size: 4

Ingredients:

- 1 small whole, boneless chicken
- 1 cup of toasted almonds
- 2 tablespoons of salted almond cream
- 1 tablespoon of pine nuts
- 2 ounces of asparagus
- a drizzle of oil

Directions:

In a large saucepan, put the chicken with a drizzle of water and oil, and cook with a lid for 15 minutes per side. Add the asparagus tips. In a bowl, prepare the dressing by putting the almond cream, almonds, and pine nuts. When the chicken is ready, spread the almond sauce on top and serve hot.

Nutritional Values: Calories: 144 kcal / Carbohydrates 18g / Protein 45g / Fat 14g / Fiber 13g

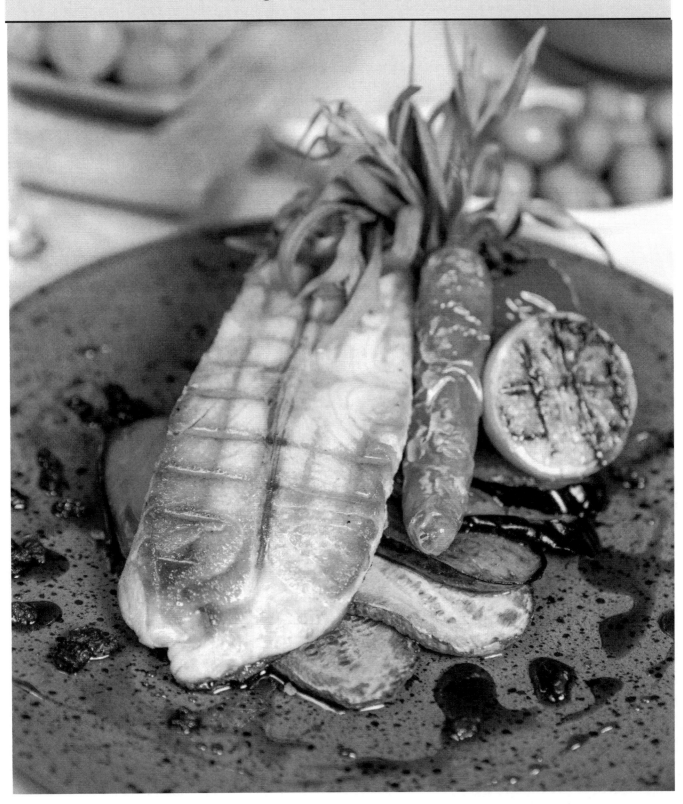

baked Sea Bass

Total time: 70 mins / **Prep Time** 15 mins / **Cooking time:** 55 mins / **Difficulty:** Easy

Serving size: 8

Ingredients:

- 8 large sea bass, clean and without entrails
- 1 lemon
- 2 sticks of rosemary
- 3 cups of potatoes, peeled and diced
- a few chopped parsley leaves
- 1 teaspoon of garlic powder
- 2 tablespoons of olive oil
- salt

Directions:

Set your oven to 390 ° F and put it on a baking sheet with a paper oven. Cut the lemon into 2 parts. The first part squeezes it for juice, and the second divides it into 8 slices. Wash the fish and put in a lemon slice for each fish. Put the pan inside and add the potatoes. Cook for 50-55 minutes or until the fish is tender. While it cooks, prepare the sauce by placing the parsley with the garlic powder and the oil in a small glass bowl. Add the salt and mix. When the fish is ready, sprinkle the sauce over the fish and, if desired, over the potatoes. Serve hot.

Nutritional Values: Calories: 80 kcal / Carbohydrates 14g / Protein 44g / Fat 20g / Fiber 3g

Raw Tuna

Total time: 8 hours / **Prep Time** 5 mins / **Cooking time:** / **Difficulty:** Easy

Serving size: 2

Ingredients:

- 2 slices of raw tuna
- 2 lemons
- 2 tablespoons of natural oil
- a pinch of salt and black pepper
- 2 pieces of rustic bread
- 3 tablespoons of white garlic sauce

- 1 bit of chopped parsley

Directions:

Put the tuna slices in a bowl and add the lemon juice and salt. Add the water and a pinch of oil and leave to marinate overnight in the refrigerator. After the marinating time has elapsed, remove the liquids and place the fish on a plate. Add a little more oil and mix the white sauce with the parsley. Add it to your plate and serve fresh with bread.

Nutritional Values: Calories: 80 kcal / Carbohydrates 14g / Protein 44g / Fat 20g / Fiber 3g

Breaded Cod

Total time: 35 mins / **Prep Time** 10 mins / **Cooking time:** 25 mins / **Difficulty:** Easy

Serving size: 3

Ingredients:

- 3 slices of cod
- 1 egg
- 1/4 cup of breadcrumbs
- a few chopped parsley leaves
- Salt and black pepper for seasoning
- 4 large leaves of curly lettuce
- fry oil

Directions:

Break the egg into a bowl and place the crumb on a plate. Beat the egg briefly and add salt and black pepper to the crumb. Dip the fish slices first in the egg, then in the crumb. Put the oil in the pan and heat. When ready, place the fish and cook for 10-15 minutes per side. Serve the washed and dried salad leaves inside.

Alternatively, you can cook without oil in your air fryer, setting 380 ° F and cooking for 15 minutes per side.

Nutritional Values: Calories: 95 kcal / Carbohydrates 18g / Protein 38g / Fat 25g / Fiber 6g

Boiled Sea Bass

Total time: 20 mins / **Prep Time** 5 mins / **Cooking time:** 15 mins / **Difficulty:** Easy

Serving size: 5

Ingredients:

- 5 sea bass, clean and without entrails
- a few leaves of parsley
- 1 drizzle of oil
- 3 crushed cloves of garlic
- 1 lemon, cut in half

Directions:

Wash your fish and put in small lemon slices with parsley. Place the fish in a large skillet, add the garlic and water and cook over medium heat with a lid for about 15 minutes. When ready, place it on a plate, squeeze the juice from the second half of the lemon over it, and season with oil (and salt if desired). Enjoy your meal.

Nutritional Values: Calories: 76 kcal / Carbohydrates 22g / Protein 41g / Fat 17g / Fiber 4g

Smoked Salmon

Total time: 5 mins / **Prep Time** 5 mins / **Cooking time:** / **Difficulty:** Easy

Serving size: 3

Ingredients:

- 6 small slices of smoked salmon, thinly sliced
- 1 lemon
- 4 tablespoons of oil
- 1 teaspoon of garlic powder
- a few leaves of parsley
- salt

Directions:

Prepare the dressing by putting the oil in a bowl, mixing with the lemon juice, and adding the garlic and parsley. Keep stirring for a few minutes.
Place the salmon on a plate and toss it with the dressing. Serve

Nutritional Values: Calories: 99 kcal / Carbohydrates 14g / Protein 46g / Fat 35g / Fiber 6g

Alkaline Sea Bass

Total time: 30 mins / **Prep Time** 15 mins / **Cooking time:** 15 mins / **Difficulty:** Easy

Serving size: 6

Ingredients:

- 3 large sea bass, clean and without entrails
- 1 avocado, peeled and seeded
- 2 boiled potatoes without peel
- 1 tablespoon of chives
- 3 crushed cloves of garlic
- 2 ounces of basil
- salt

Directions:

Wash the fish and put them in a pan. Add a drizzle of water and cook with a lid and over low heat for about 15 minutes. Make your dressing by placing the avocado, potato, and basil in a food processor. Blend for a few seconds, and then add the chives and garlic. When the fish is cooked, place it on a plate and serve with the sauce.
If the garlic flavor is too strong, you can think about putting it in the pan instead and cooking it with the fish.

Nutritional Values: Calories: 80 kcal / Carbohydrates 16g / Protein 39g / Fat 28g / Fiber 8g

Sea Salad

Total time: 55 mins / **Prep Time** 35 mins / **Cooking time:** 20 mins / **Difficulty:** Easy

Serving size: 8

Ingredients:

- 4 clean squid
- 1/2 cup of shelled clams
- 1 large octopus
- 1/2 lemon
- 3 cans of tuna in oil
- 3 cloves of garlic
- a few leaves of parsley
- 2 tablespoons of raw corn oil
- a pinch of salt

Directions:

Wash the squid and clams thoroughly and put them in a saucepan with water and salt. Bring to a boil and cook for about 20 minutes. In a second pot, put the octopus with the lemon cut into wedges, add the water and bring to a boil. Cook it for 15-20 minutes or until tender. While the fish are cooking, prepare your dressing by finely braising the garlic and parsley and mixing them with a pinch of salt. When the fish are ready, drain and place them in a large bowl, cut the octopus into small pieces and discard the head. Add the canned tuna and finish with the corn oil. Season with salt and serve cold.

Nutritional Values: Calories: 112 kcal / Carbohydrates 22g / Protein 45g / Fat 19g / Fiber 6g

Pasta with Seafood

Total time: 30 mins / **Prep Time** 15 mins / **Cooking time:** 15 mins / **Difficulty:** Easy

Serving size: 5

Ingredients:

- 2 cups of pasta
- 1 pound of clams
- 2 squid
- 3 curls, cleaned and peeled and cooked
- 2 red crabs, cleaned and cooked
- 2 cans of tuna in oil
- salt
- capers and black pepper to season

Directions:

Wash your fish thoroughly. In a large saucepan, put the water with the salt. Add the squid and clams and bring to a boil over medium heat. When it boils, drop the pasta and cook for about 15 minutes. When cooked, drain everything and put it in a bowl. Add the orange urchin eggs and the crab meat. Complete with the tuna and season with the capers and black pepper. Season with salt and serve hot.

Nutritional Values: Calories: 98 kcal / Carbohydrates 39g / Protein 38g / Fat 22g / Fiber 3g

Boiled Octopus

Total time: 50 mins / **Prep Time** 15 mins / **Cooking time:** 35 mins / **Difficulty:** Easy

Serving size: 6

Ingredients:

- 1 large octopus
- 1 cup of champignon mushrooms
- 5 medium potatoes, peeled and cut into cubes

- 2 tablespoons of chopped parsley
- 2 ounces of palm oil
- 1 teaspoon of garlic powder
- 1 teaspoon of Italian dressing
- 1 teaspoon of onion powder
- salt

Directions:

Put the octopus in a large pot, add water and salt and bring to a boil. Cook for 30-35 minutes over low heat with the lid on. Stir occasionally. In a pan, prepare the mushrooms. Cut them into slices and put them in with the potatoes. Add the parsley and a drizzle of water. Cook for about 20 minutes. When finished, put them in a bowl and wait for the octopus to be ready. Drain the water and cut it into small 1/2-inch pieces, headless. Mix it with the mushrooms and potatoes. Complete your dish by adding the Italian dressing, garlic, and onion powder. Season with salt and serve hot.

Nutritional Values: Calories: 84 kcal / Carbohydrates 33g / Protein 36g / Fat 12g / Fiber 6g

Baked Squid

Total time: 65 mins / **Prep Time** 15 mins / **Cooking time:** 50 mins / **Difficulty:** Easy

Serving size: 10

Ingredients:

- 20 giant squid clean and without entrails
- a few leaves of parsley
- 2 ounces of raw oil
- 1 teaspoon of garlic powder
- 1 lemon, squeezed

Directions:

Wash your squid thoroughly and set the oven to 385 ° F. Line a baking sheet with parchment and place your cleaned squid inside. Cook for about 45-50 minutes. While it cooks, prepare your dressing by putting the parsley, garlic powder, and oil in a bowl. Squeeze half a lemon and grate part of the peel. Mix. When the squid is ready, put them on a plate and season with the prepared sauce using a silicone marker. Serve the other half of the lemon on the scale, making small slices.

Nutritional Values: Calories: 85 kcal /

Carbohydrates 22g / Protein 38g / Fat 18g / Fiber 3g

Rocket Fish

Total time: 30 mins / **Prep Time** 10 mins / **Cooking time:** 20 mins / **Difficulty:** Easy

Serving size: 2

Ingredients:

- 1 whole sea bass, without entrails
- 1 cup of rocket leaves
- 1/2 cup cooked corn
- 1/4 cup of bean sprouts
- 1/2 lemon, cut into slices
- 2 whole and peeled cloves of garlic
- a few leaves of parsley washed
- salt

Directions:

With a knife, cut the fish lengthwise and put a few slices of lemon inside. Place the fish in a pan and add the water and the garlic cloves. Bring to a boil and cook with the lid on for 20 minutes over low heat. Cut the vegetables as you like in a large bowl and add the bean sprouts and cooked corn. When the fish is ready, cut it into 2 parts, remove the bones and serve it on 2 plates

with the vegetables. Add the parsley and add salt if you wish. Serve cool.

Nutritional Values: Calories: 77 kcal / Carbohydrates 24g / Protein 39g / Fat 11g / Fiber 24g

Roasted Salmon

Total time: 20 mins / **Prep Time** 5 mins / **Cooking time:** 15 mins / **Difficulty:** Easy

Serving size: 4

Ingredients:

- 4 slices of raw salmon
- 1/2 onion, finely chopped
- 1/2 cup black olives, without seeds
- 2 ounces of butter
- salt

Directions:

In a pan, melt the butter over medium heat, add the onion and cook for a few minutes. When they start to brown, add the salmon slices and cook for 5-10 minutes per side. When it is golden brown and crunchy, turn off the heat and serve on a plate with the olives.

Nutritional Values: Calories: 102 kcal / Carbohydrates 13g / Protein 44g / Fat 25g / Fiber 4g

CHAPTER 14: MEAT RECIPES

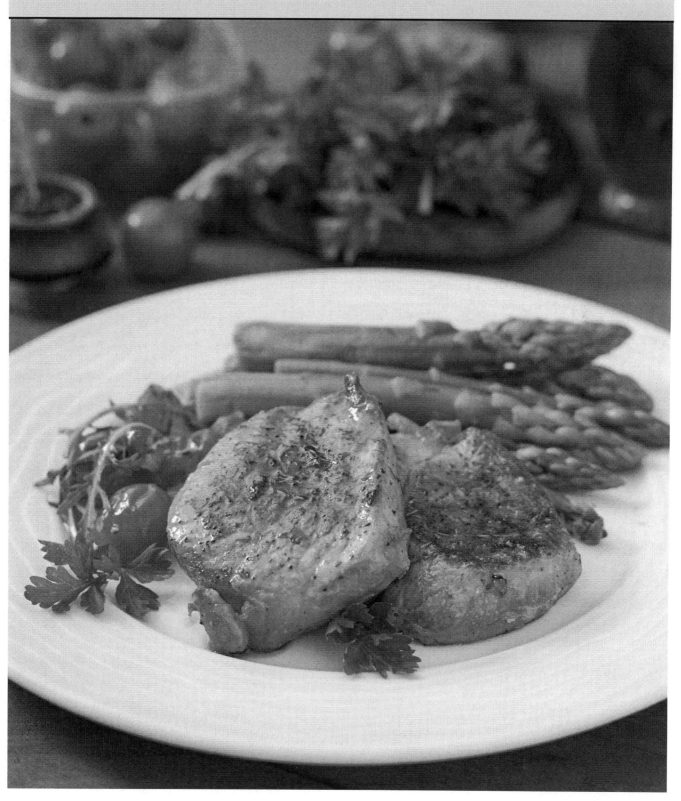

Simple Veal

Total time: 25 mins / **Prep Time** 5 mins / **Cooking time:** 20 mins / **Difficulty:** Easy

Serving size: 5

Ingredients:

- 5 slices of veal, tender and fat-free
- 3 tablespoons of oil
- 1 teaspoon of chives
- 1 teaspoon of garlic powder
- 1 bunch of green lettuce
- 1/2 cup of cherry tomatoes
- 1 tablespoon of capers

Directions:

Heat a pan and add the slices of meat when it is hot. Cook for about 10 minutes on each side. Meanwhile, prepare the sauce by putting the vegetables and tomatoes in a bowl. Add the capers and chives. Season with garlic powder. When the meat is ready, add a drizzle of raw oil and season with salt. Serve with the salad.
Nutritional Values: Calories: 95 kcal / Carbohydrates 4g / Protein 39g / Fat 3g / Fiber 19g

Sweet and sour rabbit

Total time: 65 mins / **Prep Time** 15 mins / **Cooking time:** 50 mins / **Difficulty:** Easy

Serving size: 6

Ingredients:

- 1 large rabbit
- 3 carrots, peeled and shredded
- 1 yellow pepper, finely chopped
- 1 peeled potato
- 4 finely chopped tomatoes
- salt
- black pepper for seasoning
- 1 onion, finely chopped

Directions:

In a large saucepan, put the tomatoes with the potato and pepper. Add the onion and carrots and fill with 1/2 cup of the sauce. Bring to a boil and cook for a few minutes. Next, add the raw rabbit and put the lid on. Cook over low heat for about 45-50 minutes. In the end, add salt and black pepper and serve.
Nutritional Values: Calories: 95 kcal / Carbohydrates 4g / Protein 39g / Fat 3g / Fiber 19g

Pork Stew

Total time: 1 hours / **Prep Time** 20 mins / **Cooking time:** 110 mins / **Difficulty:** Easy

Serving size: 8

Ingredients:

- 2 pounds of pork, cut into cubes
- 6 carrots, cut into small slices
- 3 medium potatoes, peeled and cut into cubes
- 3 tablespoons of oil
- 1 teaspoon of onion powder
- 1 tablespoon of chives
- salt

Directions:

Add the meat and water to a large saucepan and the potatoes and carrots. Bring to a boil and cook over low heat with the lid on for 1 hour and a half. After this time, add the onion powder and chives, cook for another 20 minutes and let it rest. Season with salt and oil and serve. Eating the next day is even better.
Nutritional Values: Calories: 114 kcal / Carbohydrates 22g / Protein 40g / Fat 14g / Fiber 8g

Roasted Veal

Total time: 5 mins / **Prep Time** 5 mins / **Cooking time:** 30 mins / **Difficulty:** Easy

Serving size: 3

Ingredients:

- 3 slices of veal
- 1 onion, cooked and finely chopped
- 2 tablespoons of oil
- 1 teaspoon of chives
- 1 teaspoon of garlic powder
- salt

Directions:

Put your slices of meat in your air fryer and cook 15 minutes per side at 390 ° F. While cooking, prepare your dressing by mixing the oil with the chives, garlic powder, and salt in a bowl. When the meat is ready, put the seasoning on top. Serve on the plate with the hot onion.

Nutritional Values: Calories: 90 kcal / Carbohydrates 4g / Protein 38g / Fat 8g / Fiber 3g

Baked Rabbit

Total time: 55 mins / **Prep Time** 5 mins / **Cooking time:** 50 mins / **Difficulty:** Easy

Serving size: 5

Ingredients:

- 1 large rabbit
- 3 cups of potatoes, peeled and cut into cubes or slices
- 1 stalk of celery
- a few leaves of parsley
- 2 teaspoons of oregano
- 1 drizzle of oil
- salt

Directions:

Set your oven to 385 ° F and line a baking sheet with parchment paper. Place the rabbit on top and the potatoes around it. Place in the oven and cook for about 50 minutes or until the meat is tender. In a food processor, blend the celery and parsley. Add the salt and a drizzle of oil and mix again. When the rabbit is almost ready, add the pureed celery to the pan and let it brown for a few minutes in the oven. Serve hot.

Nutritional Values: Calories: 95 kcal / Carbohydrates 14g / Protein 42g / Fat 12g / Fiber 6g

Veal with alkaline Seasonings

Total time: 40 mins / **Prep Time** 10 mins / **Cooking time:** 30 mins / **Difficulty:** Easy

Serving size: 2

Ingredients:

- 2 slices of veal, fat-free
- 1 avocado
- 1 potato

- 1/2 green pepper
- 1 teaspoon of chives
- 1 ounce of butter, melted
- salt

Directions:

Put the meat in a pan and cook with a bit of water and a lid for 30 minutes. In a blender, mix the avocado with the potato and pepper. Add the chives and butter with a pinch of salt. Blend until you get a homogeneous and dense mixture. When the meat is well done, serve on the plate with the freshly prepared sauce.

Nutritional Values: Calories: 80 kcal / Carbohydrates 18g / Protein 42g / Fat 3g / Fiber 11g

Baked Pork

Total time: 70 mins / **Prep Time** 10 mins / **Cooking time:** 60 mins / **Difficulty:** Easy

Serving size: 8

Ingredients:

- 3 pounds of pork, cut into large cubes
- 2 cups of potatoes, peeled and diced
- 1 onion, finely chopped
- 2 tablespoons of rosemary
- 1 teaspoon of oregano
- salt
- oil for seasoning

Directions:

Set your oven to 400 ° F and line a baking sheet with parchment paper. Place the potatoes first and then the pork. Add a drizzle of oil and the onion and cook for about 60 minutes. Give it a stir about every 20 minutes. When finished, season with oregano and rosemary. Season with salt and serve hot.

Nutritional Values: Calories: 112 kcal / Carbohydrates 23g / Protein 38g / Fat 13g / Fiber 3g

Boiled Veal

Total time: 25 mins / **Prep Time** 5 mins / **Cooking time:** 20 mins / **Difficulty:** Easy

Serving size: 3

Ingredients:

- 3 slices of veal without fat
- 3 tomatoes cut into 4 parts
- 1 ounce of green lettuce
- 1/2 cup cooked corn
- salt

Directions:

In a saucepan, put the meat and a drizzle of water. Cook over low heat with the lid for about 20 minutes. Prepare the dressing by putting the tomatoes and lettuce in a bowl, adding the corn, and seasoning with salt. When the meat is ready, serve everything on a plate.
Nutritional Values: Calories: 78 kcal / Carbohydrates 29g / Protein 41g / Fat 2g / Fiber 26g

Pork with Green Sauce

Total time: 40 mins / **Prep Time** 10 mins / **Cooking time:** 30 mins / **Difficulty:** Easy

Serving size: 5

Ingredients:

- 2.5 pounds of pork, cut into cubes
- 1 avocado
- 2 boiled potatoes without peel
- 2 boiled eggs without a shell
- 1 teaspoon of chives
- 1 teaspoon of onion powder
- salt
- 1 onion
- 2 ounces of oil
- 1/2 cup of white wine vinegar

Directions:

Make a quick sauté with the onion, oil, and salt in a saucepan. As soon as the onion begins to brown, add the pork and a drizzle of water. Cook for about 30 minutes. Add the vinegar and raise the heat when the meat is almost ready. While the meat is cooking, prepare the sauce. Put the peeled and seedless avocado in a blender and add the potatoes and eggs. Season with chives and onion powder, and season with salt. Blend until you get a nice homogeneous mixture. When the meat is ready, place it on a plate and serve with the freshly prepared sauce.

Nutritional Values: Calories: 119 kcal / Carbohydrates 32g / Protein 43g / Fat 18g / Fiber 14g

Baked Turkey

Total time: 80 mins / **Prep Time** 20 mins / **Cooking time:** 60 mins / **Difficulty:** Easy

Serving size: 7

Ingredients:

- 1 large turkey
- 3 carrots, peeled
- 4 potatoes, peeled and cut into cubes
- 1 red pepper, thinly sliced
- 1 ounce of butter
- 1 teaspoon of chives
- 1 teaspoon of Italian condiment
- 1 teaspoon of garlic powder
- 3 cups of potatoes, peeled and sliced

Directions:

Preheat the oven to 380 ° F and prepare a large baking sheet lined with parchment paper. In a food processor, put the carrots with the potatoes, and add the pepper and the butter. Season with the chives, Italian dressing, and garlic powder. Blend coarsely for a few seconds. Fill your turkey with the prepared sauce and close with string. Bake in the pan with the potatoes cut into slices. Cook for about 60 minutes. Serve hot
Nutritional Values: Calories: 140 kcal / Carbohydrates 12g / Protein 41g / Fat 24g / Fiber 4g

Meat with peppers

Total time: 50 mins / **Prep Time** 20 mins / **Cooking time:** 30 mins / **Difficulty:** Easy

Serving size: 5

Ingredients:

- 3 pounds of veal, thinly sliced and fat-free
- 1 green pepper
- 1 yellow pepper
- 1 red pepper
- 1 onion, thinly sliced
- 1/2 cup of white wine vinegar

- 1/4 cup of sugar
- salt

Directions:

In a small saucepan, cook the meat with a drizzle of water and a lid. Cook for about 25-30 minutes. In a second casserole, cook peppers, peel them and, cut them into slices not too thick, remove the seeds. Add the water and vinegar and cook for about 20 minutes. Finally, add the sugar and mix. When the meat is ready, transfer it to the saucepan with the peppers, add a drizzle of salt to season and serve hot.

Nutritional Values: Calories: 80 kcal / Carbohydrates 14g / Protein 40g / Fat 8g / Fiber 38g

Goat with eggplant

Total time: 3 hours / **Prep Time** 10 mins / **Cooking time:** 40 mins / **Difficulty:** Easy

Serving size: 6

Ingredients:

- 2 large eggplants
- 2-ounce crumbled goat cheese
- 3 tablespoons of finely chopped soft cheese
- 4 tablespoons of black olives, without seeds
- a few leaves of parsley
- 1 tablespoon of chives, finely chopped
- chopped pistachios
- salt

Directions:

Cut the aubergines into thin strips. Place them in a large, well-ordered bowl, fill them with water and salt, and press lightly. Leave to soak for at least 2 hours. Drain the water and place the aubergines on a baking tray with a paper oven. Top with olives with parsley and season with chives. In a second bowl, mix the cheeses and sprinkle them over the eggplant. Finally, put the chopped pistachios in the oven at 380 ° F for about 35-40 minutes. Serve hot or at room temperature.

Nutritional Values: Calories: 103 kcal / Carbohydrates 18g / Protein 28g / Fat 9g / Fiber 41g

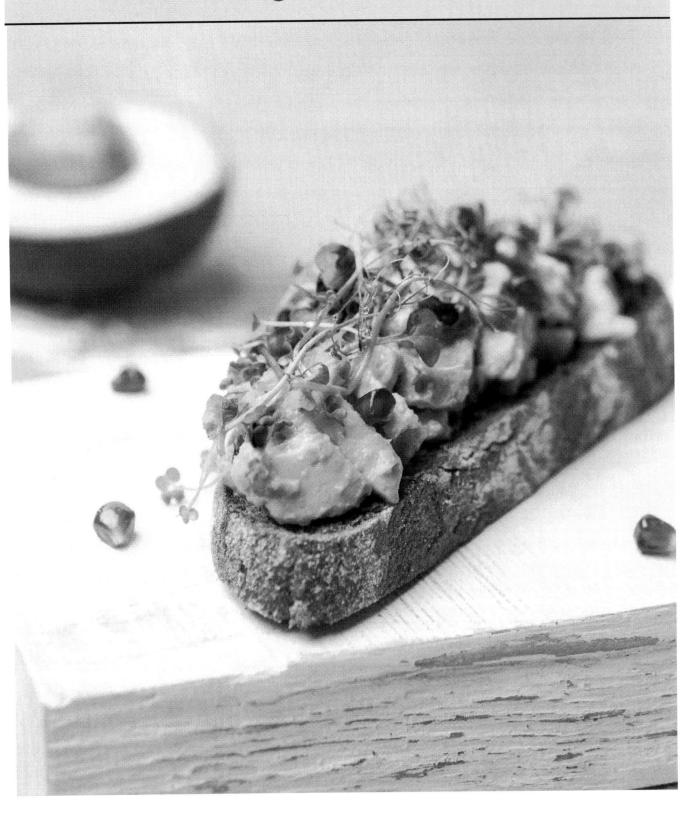

Detox Dried Fruit with Chestnut Honey

Total time: 10 mins / **Prep Time** 10 mins / **Cooking time:** / **Difficulty:** Easy

Serving size: 3

Ingredients:

- 1/2 cup of shelled walnuts
- 1/2 cup of cashews
- 1 cup of shelled almonds
- 1/4 cup of peanuts
- 3 tablespoons of chestnut honey, liquid, and brown
- 1/2 cup of blackberries

Directions:

Put all the dried fruit in a blender and blend for about 20 seconds. Transfer the chopped fruit into 3 large glasses and add the washed blackberries and honey to each one. Cold nights
Nutritional Values: Calories: 95 kcal / Carbohydrates 2g / Protein 28g / Fat 30g / Fiber 35g

Chia Breadstick and cracker

Total time: 10 mins / **Prep Time** 10 mins / **Cooking time:** / **Difficulty:** Easy

Serving size: 3

Ingredients:

- 2 cups of flour
- 1 cup of water
- 4 tablespoons of oil
- 2 ounces of chia seeds
- salt
- 1 teaspoon of yeast

To garnish

- Semolina
- Coarse salt
- oil to brush over the crackers

Directions:

Mix the flour with water, chia seeds, oil, and salt in a bowl. Create a smooth and soft dough. Spread it on a sheet of parchment paper and try to get a square and thin shape. Cut the dough with a knife, re-knead the scraps, and repeat the operation. With a fork, prick the dough so it won't swell during cooking. Add a drizzle of oil on the surface and the salt. Bake in a preheated oven at 395 ° F for about 20 minutes. Serve or store in an airless bag.
Nutritional Values: Calories: 88 kcal / Carbohydrates 32g / Protein 11g / Fat 2g / Fiber 18g

Orange and Pumpkin Salad

Total time: 25 mins / **Prep Time** 10 mins / **Cooking time:** 15 mins / **Difficulty:** Easy

Serving size: 5

Ingredients:

- 1/2 pumpkin, seedless, peeled, and cut into cubes
- 2 oranges, cut into wedges and then into 3 parts
- 1 teaspoon of not too spicy red pepper (optional)
- 1 ounce of oil
- salt and black pepper

Directions:

Put the pumpkin in a saucepan and cook for 15 minutes with a drizzle of water and lid. When finished, mix it in a bowl with the oranges. Season with oil, salt, and pepper; if you wish, add the chili. Serve fresh.
Nutritional Values: Calories: 72 kcal / Carbohydrates 38g / Protein 9g / Fat 1g / Fiber 29g

Strawberry Salad

Total time: 25 mins / **Prep Time** 10 mins / **Cooking time:** / **Difficulty:** Easy

Serving size: 10

Ingredients:

- 2.5 pounds of strawberries, washed and without green stalks
- Juice of 1 orange
- 1/4 lemon squeezed
- 1 tablespoon of sugar (or 1 teaspoon of stevia)

- 1 apple, peeled and cut into cubes
- 1 pear, peeled and cut into cubes
- 1/2 melon, seedless and cut into cubes

Directions:

Cut the strawberries in half in a large bowl, add the apple and pear, and mix. Next, add the melon and lemon. Leave to rest for about 15 minutes in the refrigerator, and finally add the orange juice. Serve cold.

Nutritional Values: Calories: 114 kcal / Carbohydrates 22g / Protein 3g / Fat 3g / Fiber 27g

Biscuits bars

Total time: 25 mins / **Prep Time** 10 mins / **Cooking time:** / **Difficulty:** Easy

Serving size: 10

Ingredients:

- 1/3 cup of butter
- 1 cup of sugar
- 2 large eggs
- 1 and 1/2 cup of flour
- yeast
- 1 ounce of milk

Directions:

Preheat the oven to 375 ° F and line a baking sheet with parchment paper. With the kitchen whisk, whip the butter and sugar. Add the eggs, and finally, add the flour with the baking powder. Keep stirring, and then add the milk. Place it in the pan and cook for about 30 minutes or until a toothpick comes out of the dough cleanly. Let it cool and serve

Nutritional Values: Calories: 120 kcal / Carbohydrates 38g / Protein 27g / Fat 3g / Fiber 2g

Chickpea Humus

Total time: 20 mins / **Prep Time** 20 mins / **Cooking time:** / **Difficulty:** Easy

Serving size: 6

Ingredients:

- 2 cups of cooked chickpeas
- 10 stalks of celery, thin

- 2 cloves of garlic (optional)
- 1 teaspoon of chives
- 1 teaspoon of garlic powder
- a pinch of black pepper
- 3 ounces of oil

Directions:

Put the chickpeas with the garlic cloves in a blender, add the oil and blend until smooth. Add the chives and garlic powder and season with black pepper. Blend for a few seconds to mix all the ingredients well. Serve at the table in a bowl, and in a second bowl, put the celery stalks, washed.

Nutritional Values: Calories: 80 kcal / Carbohydrates 41g / Protein 41g / Fat 9g / Fiber 19g

Pear and Apple Extract

Total time: 3 hours / **Prep Time** 10 mins / **Cooking time:** / **Difficulty:** Easy

Serving size: 4

Ingredients:

- 2 apples
- 2 pears
- 1 ounce of ginger
- 1/4 cup of water

Directions:

Cut the apples and pears into 4 parts, removing the peel and seeds. Next, peel the ginger and wash it quickly. Put all the fruit in the extractor and finally add the ginger. Dilute slightly with water and keep in the fridge for at least 3 hours before serving.

Nutritional Values: Calories: 50 kcal / Carbohydrates 28g / Protein 4g / Fat 0g / Fiber 18g

Fermented Zucchini

Total time: 3 days / **Prep Time** 15 mins / **Cooking time:** / **Difficulty:** Easy

Serving size: 8

Ingredients:

- 6 courgettes, cut into thin slices
- 3% brine
- Peel 1 red apple

Directions:

Prepare the brine with 2 cups of water and 1/4 teaspoon of salt and stir. Place the sliced zucchini in a glass bowl and add pieces of apple peel. Fill the bowl with the brine and close; keep in the fridge. After 2 days, the zucchini starts to ferment; if a bit of liquid comes out, it is average, clean with a cloth. On the third day, your courgettis are ready to be enjoyed. Store in the refrigerator for up to 20 days.
Nutritional Values: Calories: 35 kcal / Carbohydrates 18g / Protein 2g / Fat 0g / Fiber 41g

Purifying Juice

Total time: 10 mins / **Prep Time** 10 mins / **Cooking time:** / **Difficulty:** Easy

Serving size: 4

Ingredients:

- 1 avocado
- 1 peeled apple
- 1 peeled kiwi
- 1 peeled pear
- 1/3 lemon without peel
- 1 inch of ginger, peeled
- 1/2 cup of green grapes
- 1/3 of yellow mango
- 1 vanilla pod

- 1 pinch of salt

Directions:

Put all the fruit in a food processor and blend. Filter the juice and infuse the vanilla stick for a few minutes. Drink immediately, adding a pinch of salt first.
Nutritional Values: Calories: 80 kcal / Carbohydrates 10g / Protein 3g / Fat 0g / Fiber 25g

Avocado Salad

Total time: 20 mins / **Prep Time** 20 mins / **Cooking time:** / **Difficulty:** Easy

Serving size: 6

Ingredients:

- 3 avocados, seedless and peeled
- 1 head of pureed green cabbage
- 1 lettuce, chopped
- 3 medium tomatoes, cut into 4 parts
- 1 teaspoon of capers
- raw oil

Directions:

Mix the cabbage with the lettuce in a large bowl and add the tomatoes and chopped avocado. Season with the capers and a drizzle of oil. Serve fresh.
Nutritional Values: Calories: 102 kcal / Carbohydrates 19g / Protein 9g / Fat 4g / Fiber 37g

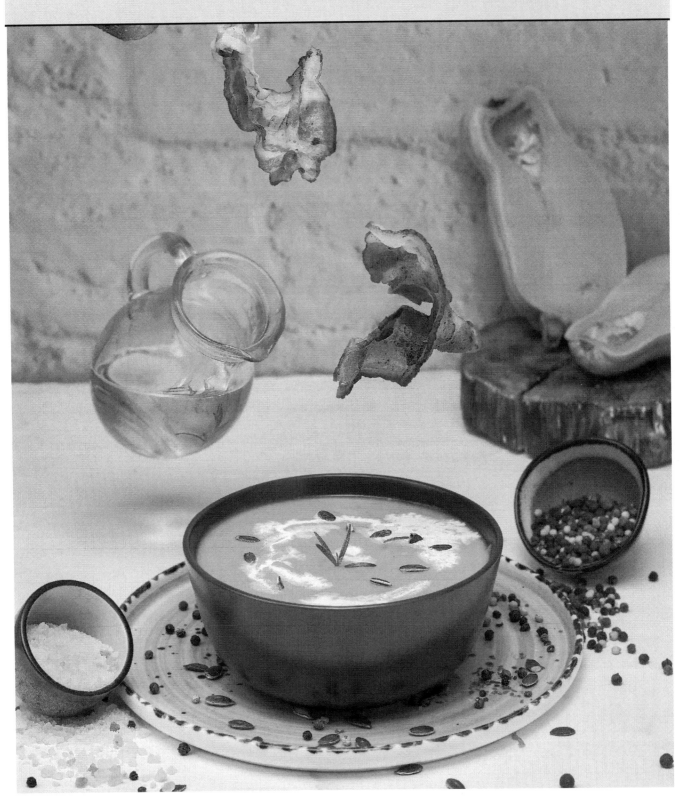

Garlic soup

Total time: 75 mins / **Prep Time** 10 mins / **Cooking time:** 60 mins / **Difficulty:** Easy

Serving size: 12

Ingredients:

- 10 cloves of garlic, crushed
- 3 potatoes, peeled
- 1 tablespoon of processed flour
- 2 large carrots
- 1 ounce of butter
- 1 teaspoon of the vegetable cube
- salt
- 1 teaspoon of garlic powder
- 1 tablespoon of Italian dressing
- 1 teaspoon of hot pepper (optional)

Directions:

In a saucepan, make a quick sauté with garlic and butter. As soon as the garlic turns golden, fill your pan 3/4 full and add the finely chopped potatoes and flour. Bring to a boil and cook over low heat with a lid. Next, add the carrots and the cube. After 40 minutes of cooking, add the rest of the ingredients, and if you like spicy, add the chili too. Finally, season with salt and serve. If you wish, remove the garlic cloves and drink the hot broth. You can also store it in the refrigerator for 6 days in an airtight container.

Nutritional Values: Calories: 89 kcal / Carbohydrates 18g / Protein 8g / Fat 6g / Fiber 19g

Onion Soup

Total time: 70 mins / **Prep Time** 10 mins / **Cooking time:** 60 mins / **Difficulty:** Easy

Serving size: 8

Ingredients:

- 4 large onions, peeled and cut into 4 parts
- 1 tablespoon of curry
- 1 tablespoon of the vegetable cube
- 1 tablespoon of processed flour
- 4 medium potatoes, peeled
- 2 carrots
- salt
- 1 teaspoon of onion powder
- 1 tablespoon of Italian dressing
- 1 drizzle of oil

Directions:

In a saucepan, make a quick sauté with the oil and onions. When the onions begin to brown, fill with water and bring to a boil. When it boils, lower the heat and add the flour with the very finely chopped potatoes. Add the carrots and the cube. Cook for 40 minutes. Add the Italian dressing, onion powder, and curry. Continue cooking for another 20 minutes and serve hot. You can also refrigerate for up to 5 days in a closed container.

Nutritional Values: Calories: 94 kcal / Carbohydrates 19g / Protein 12g / Fat 4g / Fiber 22g

Pepper Soup

Total time: 75 mins / **Prep Time** 15 mins / **Cooking time:** 60 mins / **Difficulty:** Easy

Serving size: 6

Ingredients:

- 2 yellow peppers
- 1 green pepper
- 1 red pepper
- 2 ounces of butter
- 1 large onion, peeled and finely chopped
- 1 teaspoon of garlic powder
- 1 tablespoon of Italian dressing
- 1 tablespoon of processed flour
- salt

Directions:

Finely chop all the peppers, be sure to remove the green stalk and remove the internal seeds if you wish. Put the onion with the butter in a large saucepan and make a quick sauté. When the onion begins to brown, add the water and bring it to a boil. Add the peppers and flour. Cook with the lid on for at least 40 minutes. Then add the Italian dressing and garlic powder and cook for another 20 minutes or so or until the peppers are tender. Serve hot.

Nutritional Values: Calories: 102 kcal /

Carbohydrates 18g / Protein 16g / Fat 9g / Fiber 32g

Green Soup

Total time: 70 mins / **Prep Time** 20 mins / **Cooking time:** 50 mins / **Difficulty:** Easy

Serving size: 10

Ingredients:

- 2 green peppers
- 1 stalk of celery
- 2 bay leaves
- 1 onion
- 2 potatoes, finely chopped and peeled
- 1 teaspoon of the vegetable cube
- salt

Directions:

Put the celery, bay leaves, water, and salt in a large pot, and bring to a boil. While heating the water, cut the pepper into thin strips and put it in the pool. Add the finely chopped onion, stock cube, and potatoes when it boils. Cook for about 50 minutes and turn off and serve.
Nutritional Values: Calories: 78 kcal / Carbohydrates 12g / Protein 14g / Fat 2g / Fiber 36g

cheeses Soup

Total time: 70 mins / **Prep Time** 10 mins / **Cooking time:** 60 mins / **Difficulty:** Easy

Serving size: 5

Ingredients:

- 1 ounce of soft cheese cubes
- 1 ounce of shredded hard cheese
- 2 ounces of aged Parmesan, grated
- 3 ounces of drained mozzarella
- 2 potatoes, peeled
- 1 tablespoon of flour
- salt and black pepper for seasoning
- 1 teaspoon of chives

Directions:

In a large bowl, prepare the first 3 kinds of cheese by mixing them. Add a pinch of black pepper to flavor them and the chives. Cook the finely chopped potatoes in a saucepan with flour and water. Bring to a boil and lower the heat. Cook for 30 minutes. Add the cheeses except for mozzarella and continue cooking for another 60 minutes. When done, serve hot and add the mozzarella. This way, the cheese will eventually melt and become stringy. Serve hot.
Nutritional Values: Calories: 98 kcal / Carbohydrates 19g / Protein 24g / Fat 19g / Fiber 3g

Boiled Vegetables Soup

Total time: 45 mins / **Prep Time** 5 mins / **Cooking time:** 40 mins / **Difficulty:** Easy

Serving size: 9

Ingredients:

- 1 bunch of green lettuce
- 1 red pepper, thinly sliced and seedless
- 1 yellow pepper, thinly sliced and seedless
- 1 bay leaf
- 1 stalk of celery
- 2 potatoes, peeled and finely chopped
- 1 onion, peeled and finely chopped
- 1 bunch of curly lettuce
- salt
- 1 tablespoon of Italian dressing

Directions:

In a large saucepan, put the peppers and salt, add the water and bring to a boil. Cook for about 20 minutes over low heat and with a lid. Then add the green lettuce, celery, potatoes, and onion with the curly lettuce. Continue cooking for 10 minutes, and then add the bay leaf. Season with Italian seasoning and season with salt. Serve hot or refrigerate for up to 8 days.
Nutritional Values: Calories: 70 kcal / Carbohydrates 15g / Protein 17g / Fat 1g / Fiber 28g

Spinach Soup

Total time: 40 mins / **Prep Time** 10 mins / **Cooking time:** 30 mins / **Difficulty:** Easy

Serving size: 8

Ingredients:

- 3 pounds of fresh spinach

- 3 cloves of garlic
- 3 ounces of butter
- 1/2 onion, finely chopped and peeled
- 2 potatoes, peeled
- 1 tablespoon of Italian dressing
- salt

Directions:

In a saucepan, make a quick sauté with the butter and garlic. Add the onion and mix. Cook for a few minutes on high heat. When the garlic and onion begin to brown, add the water, potatoes, and spinach. Bring to a boil and cook for about 30 minutes with the lid on and on a low flame. When the soup gets the desired density, turn off the heat and serve hot with a good, grated cheese.

Nutritional Values: Calories: 85 kcal / Carbohydrates 12g / Protein 20g / Fat 12g / Fiber 19g

Meat Soup

Total time: 2,5 hours / **Prep Time** 30 mins / **Cooking time:** 125 mins / **Difficulty:** Easy

Serving size: 4

Ingredients:

- 1 pound of veal, cut into pieces
- 1/2 pound of chicken meat
- 3 ounces of minced meat
- 2 ounces of chives
- 2 onions, finely chopped
- 1 tablespoon of meat cube
- 1 ounce of butter
- salt and black pepper

Directions:

In a large saucepan, sauté the onion and butter quickly, and add the chives in the sauce and a pinch of salt and black pepper. When the onion starts to brown,

put all the meat in the pan and stir quickly for a few minutes. Fill the pot with water and add the nut. Bring to a boil and cook over low heat for at least 2 hours. The meat must be tender and soft. When finished, season with salt and serve, or you can keep it in the fridge for up to 3 days.

Nutritional Values: Calories: 115 kcal / Carbohydrates 8g / Protein 45g / Fat 19g / Fiber 3g

Turnip Soup

Total time: 55 mins / **Prep Time** 10 mins / **Cooking time:** 45 mins / **Difficulty:** Easy

Serving size: 8

Ingredients:

- 2 bunches of turnips
- 3 potatoes, peeled and finely chopped
- 1 cup of pre-cooked chickpeas
- 1 stick of rosemary
- salt
- 1 teaspoon of a vegetable cube
- 1 tablespoon of flour
- salt and black pepper for seasoning
- 1 ounce of butter
- 1 cherry tomato divided into quarters

Directions:

In a saucepan, put the butter and turnips. Add the tomato and salt and cook over medium heat for a few minutes. After, add the water with the salt, the cube, potatoes and the flour and bring to a boil. Lower the heat and cook with the lid on for about 40 minutes. Towards the end of cooking, add the chickpeas and season with rosemary. Add salt and black pepper and serve with a few slices of whole meal bread.

Nutritional Values: Calories: 93 kcal / Carbohydrates 12g / Protein 18g / Fat 3g / Fiber 24g

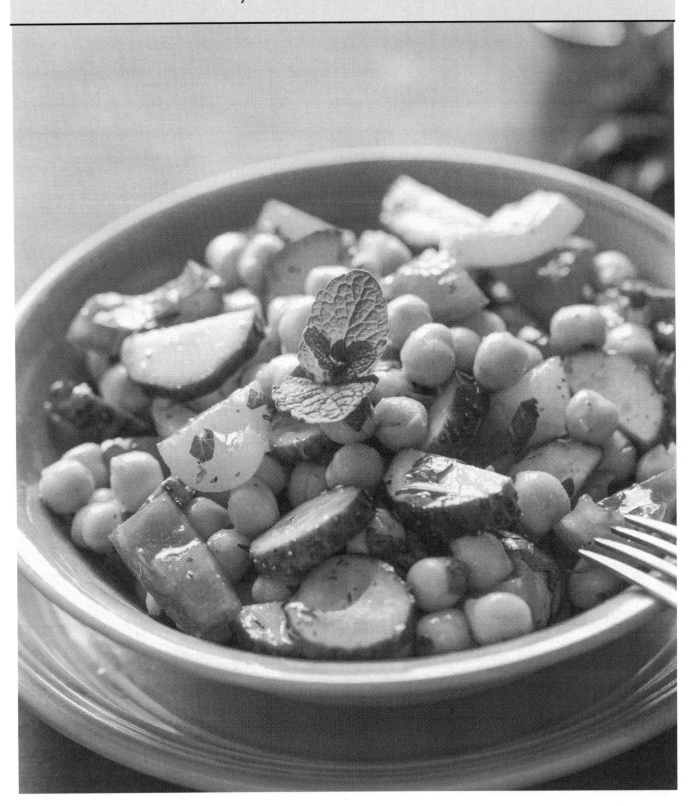

Anti-inflammatory Vegetables

Total time: Prep Time 20 mins / **Difficulty:** Easy

Serving size: 6

Ingredients:

- anti-inflammatory vegetables
- 1 stalk of celery
- 2 courgettes
- 1 small onion, peeled and cut into 8 parts
- 1 cup 3% brine

Directions:

First, prepare the brine by putting 1.5 teaspoons of salt in 1 cup of water. Stir, and your brine is ready. Next, cut the celery and the courgettes into small slices with the peel. Also, cut the onion evenly and place all the vegetables in a sterilized glass jar. Add the brine and close with the cap. Let it rest in a cool, dark place for about 5 days, and at least once a day, open the containers to let the gases escape. After 5 days, your vegetables will be fermented correctly and ready to be enjoyed. You can keep them in the refrigerator for about 20 days.

Nutritional Values: Calories: 50 kcal / Carbohydrates 32g / Protein 19g / Fat 3g / Fiber 44g

Avocado Pizza

Total time: 2 hours / **Prep Time** 30 mins / **Cooking time:** 50 mins / **Difficulty:** Medium

Serving size: 2

Ingredients:

- 1/2 cup of whole flour
- 1 avocado, peeled and unseen
- salt and black pepper
- 1 teaspoon of yeast
- 2 tablespoons of tomato sauce
- 1 ounce of soft cheese cubes
- oil for seasoning

Directions:

In a large bowl, put the flour, salt, and yeast. Cut the avocado into 2 parts, the first into slices in a bowl, the second part mash it all into a pulp and add it to the flour. Slowly begins to pour the water and knead. Knead until you get a soft and thick, non-sticky dough. Let it rise for about 60 minutes or until it doubles in size. Alternatively, you can use your mixer and not get your hands dirty. When the dough is ready, roll it out and make your pizza, sprinkle over the sauce with the cheese and sliced avocado. Bake in a hot oven at 400 ° F for about 50 minutes, wait for the cheese to melt, and serve hot with a drizzle of oil.

Nutritional Values: Calories: 140 kcal / Carbohydrates 40g / Protein 22g / Fat 6g / Fiber 3g

Anti-inflammatory Broth

Total time: 70 mins / **Prep Time** 10 mins / **Cooking time:** 60 mins / **Difficulty:** Easy

Serving size: 5

Ingredients:

- 1 large tomato
- 1 large onion and peeled
- 2 stalks of celery
- 2 potatoes, peeled and finely chopped
- 1 tablespoon of carob flour
- 1 tablespoon of Italian dressing
- 1 clove of garlic
- salt

Directions:

In a large saucepan, put the tomato with the onion and celery. Add the garlic and potatoes and leave them whole. Add the water, salt, and flour and bring to a boil. Cook over low heat for about 1 hour with the lid on. At the end of cooking, add the Italian dressing and serve.

Nutritional Values: Calories: 60 kcal / Carbohydrates 12g / Protein 2g / Fat 0g / Fiber 30g

Carrots Cream

Total time: 25 mins / **Prep Time** 5 mins / **Cooking time:** 20 mins / **Difficulty:** Easy

Serving size: 3

Ingredients:

- 5 carrots, peeled and coarsely chopped
- 2 potatoes, peeled and finely chopped
- a few leaves of parsley

- 1 teaspoon of chives

Directions:

In a saucepan, boil the potatoes and carrots with water and salt. After 20 minutes of cooking, turn off and drain. Now put the potatoes and carrots in a blender, add the seasonings and blend until pure. Keep in a bowl and serve in combination with vegetable or meat dishes.

Nutritional Values: Calories: 50 kcal / Carbohydrates 18g / Protein 2g / Fat 1g / Fiber 34g

Avocado and Eggs Salad

Total time: 20 mins / **Prep Time** 10 mins / **Cooking time:** 10 mins / **Difficulty:** Easy

Serving size: 6

Ingredients:

- 2 avocados, peeled and seeded
- 8 medium eggs
- 1 bunch of curly lettuce
- 1/2 red chard, sliced
- 1 stalk of celery, chopped
- White sauce basic for seasoning

Directions:

In a saucepan, boil the eggs for about 10 minutes with water. When finished, wait for them to cool, peel them, and cut them into 4. Wash and cut the salad in a large salad bowl and add the diced avocado and eggs. Add the chard and celery and season with the white sauce. Stir and serve.

Nutritional Values: Calories: 94 kcal / Carbohydrates 24g / Protein 8g / Fat 10g / Fiber 32g

Vegetable Cake

Total time: 100 mins / **Prep Time** 30 mins / **Cooking time:** 65 mins / **Difficulty:** Easy

Serving size: 8

Ingredients:

Cake

- 1 cup of whole meal flour
- 3 eggs
- 1/2 cup of coconut milk
- 1/4 cup of sugar

- salt for seasoning
- 1 teaspoon of yeast

Seasoning

- 2 green peppers
- 3 carrots, peeled
- 2 potatoes, peeled and finely chopped

Cream

- 1 boiled potato, peeled
- 1 peeled and seedless avocado
- salt

Directions:

Prepare the vegetables by peeling and cutting the peppers and carrots. Cook them in a pot with a bit of water and carrots for about 15 minutes. Also, make the salted avocado cream by squeezing the pulp and mixing it with the potato and salt. Finally, prepare the cake by mixing the liquid eggs with the sugar and then gradually adding the flour with the baking powder. When the dough gets too hard, add the coconut milk and a pinch of salt. Let it rest for a few minutes, then transfer it to a cake mold. Then pour the mixture, add the cooked and blended vegetables, and mix everything. Bake for about 50 minutes at 380 ° F. When well done, turn off the oven and let it cool. Cut it in half and add the prepared avocado cream. Close and serve.

Nutritional Values: Calories: 104 kcal / Carbohydrates 38g / Protein 12g / Fat 14g / Fiber 38g

Vegetables Pizza

Total time: 2 hours / **Prep Time** 20 mins / **Cooking time:** 50 mins / **Difficulty:** Easy

Serving size: 4

Ingredients:

- 2 cups of whole wheat flour
- 1 teaspoon of yeast
- salt
- 1 cup of water (approx.)
- 1 tablespoon of seed oil
- 1 green pepper
- 1/4 cup of bean sprouts
- 2 ounces of vegan cheese, diced

- 1 teaspoon of red pepper
- 1 small potato lightly cooked, peeled, and cut into cubes
- 1 cup of tomato sauce
- 2 tablespoons of oregano

Directions:

Put the flour, baking powder, and salt in a large bowl. Start mixing by adding the water gently. Knead until you get a dense and uniform paste. If it is too hard, add the oil and continue kneading. Set it aside and let it rise for at least 1 hour. In the meantime, prepare the vegetables, peel the pepper and cut it into strips, mix it with the cheese, the potato, and the chili. When the dough has risen, divide it into 4 parts and start rolling out your dough. Spread the tomato sauce and the prepared dressing. Bake in a preheated oven at 400 ° F for about 45-50 minutes. When ready, add oregano and serve

Nutritional Values: Calories: 125 kcal / Carbohydrates 36g / Protein 16g / Fat 6g / Fiber 15g

Veggie dips

Total time: 30 mins / **Prep Time** 10 mins / **Cooking time:** 20 mins / **Difficulty:** Easy

Serving size: 12

Ingredients:

- 10 carrots, peeled and cut into strips
- 1 green pepper, peeled, seeded, and cut into strips
- 1 onion, peeled and sliced
- 20 large green lettuce leaves, cut in half
- 20 large leaves of curly lettuce, cut in half
- Fry oil
- 3 large eggs
- 1/2 cup crumb

- 1 clove of garlic, peeled and finely chopped
- a few chopped parsley leaves
- salt and pepper for seasoning

Directions:

Prepare the crumb, season it with the minced garlic, salt, and pepper, add the parsley, and mix. Heat the oil in a saucepan and dip each vegetable first in the eggs and then in the seasoned crumb. Now dip the breaded vegetables in boiling oil and let each vegetable cook for 10-15 minutes; make sure it is well immersed. Drain the oil and place the vegetables in a large bowl with paper towels. Serve hot.

Nutritional Values: Calories: 100 kcal / Carbohydrates 38g / Protein 12g / Fat 15g / Fiber 40g

Tomatoes and Zucchini

Total time: 10 mins / **Prep Time** 10 mins / **Cooking time:** / **Difficulty:** Easy

Serving size: 4

Ingredients:

- 5 large tomatoes, quartered
- 3 courgettes cut into strips and then in half
- 2 tablespoons of capers
- 1 teaspoon of powdered rosemary
- 1 ounce of raw oil
- 1 tablespoon of black pepper granules
- salt

Directions:

In a large bowl, mix the tomatoes with the zucchini. Combine with capers and oil and mix. Add the black pepper and rosemary and continue mixing. Before serving, add salt and enjoy your meal.

Nutritional Values: Calories: 77 kcal / Carbohydrates 32g / Protein 8g / Fat 1g / Fiber 44g

CHAPTER 18: DESSERT RECIPES

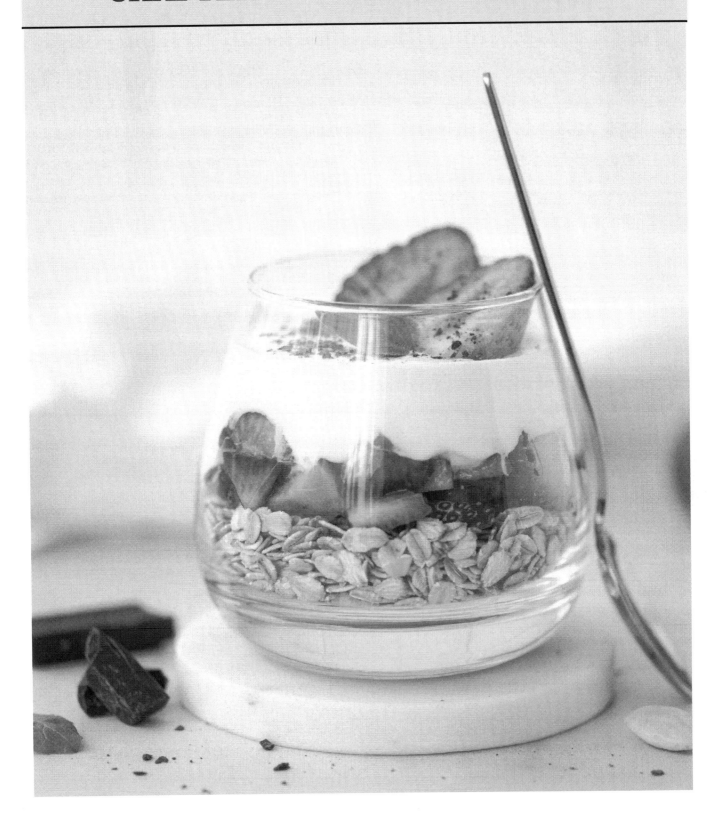

Chocolate Cookies

Total time: 60 mins / **Prep Time** 10 mins / **Cooking time:** 50 mins / **Difficulty:** Easy

Serving size: 18

Ingredients:

- 1 cup of processed flour
- 1/3 cup of sugar
- 2 medium eggs
- 2 ounces of oil
- 1/2 cup of shredded dark chocolate

Directions:

In a large bowl, mix the flour with the sugar and eggs. Help yourself with the kitchen whips. When the dough starts to get hard, add the seed oil. When the dough has reached a good density, add the chocolate and mix to complete. Let him remarry. Preheat the oven to 360 ° F and line a baking sheet with parchment paper. Cut the dough into slices and place them evenly inside the pan. Cook for about 45-50 minutes or until the biscuits dry. Serve at room temperature.
Nutritional Values: Calories: 112 kcal / Carbohydrates 30g / Protein 8g / Fat 6g / Sugar 10g

Coconut Cream Bars

Total time: 50 mins / **Prep Time** 30 mins / **Cooking time:** 20 mins / **Difficulty:** Easy

Serving size: 12

Ingredients:

- 1 cup of whole grains,
- 1 pound of 5-grain cookies
- 1/2 cup chestnut honey, liquid
- hazelnut cream to garnish
- 2 liquid eggs

Directions:

Put the cereals and biscuits in a blender. Blend coarsely. Add the eggs and mix with a spatula. Using your hands, start kneading and add the honey. This, in addition to a pleasing aroma, will allow the dough to stick. Start making a serpentine and cut it to the size you prefer. Place your bars on a plate and garnish with the hazelnut cream. Serve

Nutritional Values: Calories: 150 kcal / Carbohydrates 35g / Protein 14g / Fat 29g / Sugar 18g

Almond Cake

Total time: 70 mins / **Prep Time** 20 mins / **Cooking time:** 50 mins / **Difficulty:** Easy

Serving size: 8

Ingredients:

- 1/2 cup of almonds
- 1 cup of flour
- 1 cup of sugar
- 2 eggs
- 2 ounces of sunflower oil
- 1 pinch of salt
- 1 teaspoon of baking powder
- Powdered sugar for serving

Directions:

Prepare the almonds by soaking them in hot water. This way, the brown skin will go away. Drain and chop coarsely. Mix the eggs with the sugar in a large glass bowl first, then add the yeast and a pinch of salt. Start kneading with a whisk, adding the flour gently. Try to get a creamy and thick dough. Add the oil and continue kneading. Transfer the dough to a cake pan and add the almonds on top. Bake in a hot oven at about 325 ° F. Bake for 45-50 minutes and wait until the dough is dry. Serve with a sprinkle of powdered sugar on top.
Nutritional Values: Calories: 130 kcal / Carbohydrates 40g / Protein 18g / Fat 12g / Sugar 16g

Kiwi with Dried Fruit

Total time: 2 hours / **Prep Time** 5 mins / **Cooking time:** / **Difficulty:** Easy

Serving size: 10

Ingredients:

- 6 large kiwis
- a mix of nuts (walnuts, cashews, hazelnuts, almonds)
- 1/2 cup of natural yogurt
- 1 tablespoon of honey

Directions:

Blend the dried fruit coarsely with a food processor and set aside. Peel the kiwis and cut them into quarters in a bowl. Add the dried fruit mix and mix everything with the yogurt and honey. Let it rest for about 90 minutes in the refrigerator. In this way, the flavors blend. Serve fresh in a small bowl.

Nutritional Values: Calories: 95 kcal / Carbohydrates 20g / Protein 22g / Fat 30g / Sugar 8g Fiber 12g

Homemade Protein Bars

Total time: 25 mins / **Prep Time** 25 mins / **Cooking time:** / **Difficulty:** Easy

Serving size: 14

Ingredients:

- 2 cups of oatmeal
- 1/2 cup of grated coconut
- 1 tablespoon of stevia (or another sweetener)
- 3 ounces of melted chocolate

Directions:

In a bowl, mix the oatmeal with the coconut. Also, add the sweetener and gently put the water. Wait for the mixture to thicken and start working it with your hands. Make your own thin bars and put them on a plate. Before serving, sprinkle them with the pampered liquid and enjoy.

Nutritional Values: Calories: 135 kcal / Carbohydrates 30g / Protein 30g / Fat 35g / Sugar 14g

Banana and nuts Muffin

Total time: 1 hour / **Prep Time** 10 mins / **Cooking time:** 50 mins / **Difficulty:** Easy

Serving size: 6

Ingredients:

- 1 cup of flour
- 2 eggs
- 1 ounce of butter
- 1 cup of sugar
- 1/4 cup almond milk (approx.)
- 1 teaspoon of yeast
- 2 bananas, peeled and sliced and cut into rings
- 1/2 cup of shredded walnuts

- a pinch of salt

Directions:

First, mix the eggs with the sugar in a bowl, and then add the yeast. Start adding the flour gently and knead with the help of a whisk. Add the almond milk and butter when the dough starts to get hard. When the dough is ready, add the bananas and walnuts as well. Preheat the oven to 360 ° F and pour the batter into the muffin cups. Place them in a pan and bake for 45-50 minutes. Wait until they are scorched. Serve at room temperature.

Nutritional Values: Calories: 140 kcal / Carbohydrates 25g / Protein 10g / Fat 8g / Sugar 18g

Strawberry Jam

Total time: 1 hour / **Prep Time** 30 mins / **Cooking time:** 40 mins / **Difficulty:** Easy

Serving size: 10

Ingredients:

- 6 cups of strawberries
- 3 pounds of sugar
- 1.5 tablespoons of pectin

Directions:

Wash the strawberries thoroughly and remove the stem. Cut them into 2 parts and put them in a large saucepan. Add the sugar and mix. Finally, add the pectin and start cooking over high heat. As soon as the jam begins to simmer, stir gently without ever stopping, and when the boiling increases, lower the heat. Wait for the mixture's proper density (35-40 minutes) and turn off the heat. Put the hot jam into sterilized glass jars and when complete, seal tightly and flip. Let it cool, and then fix the pot. In this way, your spot can be stored for 24 months.

Nutritional Values: Calories: 120 kcal / Carbohydrates 20g / Protein 18g / Fat 3g / Sugar 24g

Simple Anti-inflammatory Biscuit

Total time: 55 mins / **Prep Time** 5 mins / **Cooking time:** 50 mins / **Difficulty:** Easy

Serving size: 14

Ingredients:

- 1.5 cups of whole wheat flour
- 1 cup of sugar

- 3 eggs
- 1/4 lemon zest
- 1 orange juice
- 1 ounce of corn oil
- salt

Directions:

In a bowl, mix the eggs with the sugar. Add a pinch of salt and gently start pouring the flour. Knead using the kitchen whisk. Continuing to knead, finally, add the oil and orange juice. In the end, add the lemon zest and mix for a few seconds to mix all the ingredients well. Let it rest and preheat the oven to 355 ° F. Create the shapes you want with your dough and place them in a baking tray lined with parchment. Bake for 45-50 minutes, waiting for the mixture to dry. Serve at room temperature with a good detox juice.

Nutritional Values: Calories: 77 kcal / Carbohydrates 17g / Protein 9g / Fat 6g / Sugar 11g

Cereal with Yogurt

Total time: 5 mins / **Prep Time** 5 mins / **Cooking time:** / **Difficulty:** Easy

Serving size: 4

Ingredients:

- 2 cups of yogurt
- 1 cup of whole grains
- 1/4 cup of blackberries
- 1/4 cup of red berries
- 1 teaspoon of honey
- 1 banana, cut into slices
- 1/8 cup of oats

Directions:

In a large bowl, put the red and black berries and mix them with the honey. Next, add the cereals and finally the yogurt. Mix everything and add the oats as well. Create 4 portions and serve fresh.

Nutritional Values: Calories: 65 kcal / Carbohydrates 20g / Protein 12g / Fat 3g / Sugar 2g

Coconut Chips

Total time: 20 mins / **Prep Time** 10 mins / **Cooking time:** 10 mins / **Difficulty:** Easy

Serving size: 13

Ingredients:

- 1 coconut, peeled and cut into small slices
- fry oil
- powdered sugar for seasoning

Directions:

Cut the coconut into the desired shape. In a saucepan, heat the oil, and dip the coconut slices when ready. Let them cook for about 10 minutes. When done, blot the oil with paper towels and serve hot with a sprinkle of icing sugar.

Nutritional Values: Calories: 130 kcal / Carbohydrates 18g / Protein 11g / Fat 35g / Sugar 6g

Apple Cake

Total time: 70 mins / **Prep Time** 10 mins / **Cooking time:** 60 mins / **Difficulty:** Easy

Serving size: 8

Ingredients:

- 2 cups of processed flour
- 1.5 cups of sugar
- 4 large eggs
- 3 ounces of butter
- 2 apples, peeled and thinly sliced
- 1 tablespoon of yeast
- vanillin to flavor
- a pinch of salt

Directions:

In a large bowl, prepare your dough by beating the eggs with the sugar and then gradually adding the flour with the baking powder. Help yourself with the kitchen whips. Add the butter (preferably melted) and vanilla. Add a pinch of salt, and when the dough is ready, add the sliced apples. Preheat the oven to 350 ° F and pour the batter into your favorite cake pan. Cook for 50-60 minutes or until the wrong is well done.

Nutritional Values: Calories: 140 kcal / Carbohydrates 25g / Protein 11g / Fat 12g / Sugar 16g

Coconut and Almond Biscuits

Total time: 55 mins / **Prep Time** 10 mins / **Cooking time:** 45 mins / **Difficulty:** Easy

Serving size: 10

Ingredients:

- 12 coconut, peeled and grated
- 1 cup of walnuts, chopped
- 2 cups of flour
- 1 cup of sugar
- 3 eggs
- 1 tablespoon of butter
- a pinch of salt

Directions:

Place the almonds in a baking dish and set the oven to 200 ° F. Toast them lightly for about ten minutes, the time you prepare the dough. Mix the eggs with the sugar in a bowl and add the flour. Start kneading with a whisk and add the butter. Finish by adding the salt. When your dough has the proper density, sweep the oven and mix the almonds with the coconut. Add them to the dough and finish with a pinch of salt. Mix everything and preheat the oven to 360 ° F. Place your cookies with the mold of your choice and arrange them neatly on the parchment paper of the oven rack. Cook for about 45 minutes or until cooked through. Serve at room temperature.

Nutritional Values: Calories: 150 kcal / Carbohydrates 30g / Protein 18g / Fat 20g / Sugar 21g

Apple Muffin

Total time: 45 mins / **Prep Time** 5 mins / **Cooking time:** 40 mins / **Difficulty:** Easy

Serving size: 3

Ingredients:

- 1/2 cup of flour
- 1/3 cup of sugar
- 2 eggs
- 1 tablespoon of seed oil
- 1 apple, peeled and shredded
- 1/2 lemon squeezed
- 1 teaspoon of yeast

Directions:

Put the apple with the lemon juice in a medium bowl, so it doesn't turn black. Mix the sugar with the eggs in a large bowl and gradually add the flour. Knead with a

whisk and also add the oil and yeast. Add the apples and mix everything when the dough reaches the perfect consistency. Set your oven to 350 ° F and place the dough in the muffin cups. When ready, bake for 40 minutes or until the dough is well leavened and dry.

Nutritional Values: Calories: 78 kcal / Carbohydrates 22g / Protein 7g / Fat 3g / Sugar 24g

Apple Alkaline Cream

Total time: 2 hours / **Prep Time** 15 mins / **Cooking time:** 35 mins / **Difficulty:** Easy

Serving size: 10

Ingredients:

- 6 red apples, peeled and seedless
- 2 cups of sugar
- 1/2 avocado, peeled and seeded
- 1/2 lemon squeezed
- a pinch of salt

Directions:

Place the finely chopped apples in a saucepan and add the sugar and avocado. Combine the lemon juice and salt. Start heating over medium heat and remember to stir constantly. Make sure that the avocado mixes well with the apple. Cook for about 30 minutes. Finally, put the fruit in the vegetable mash and take the pulp. Let it cool and store it in a hermetically sealed glass container. Keep in the fridge for 3 days.

Nutritional Values: Calories: 110 kcal / Carbohydrates 30g / Protein 8g / Fat 2g / Sugar 26g

Yogurt and dried Fruit

Total time: 15 mins / **Prep Time** 15 mins / **Cooking time:** / **Difficulty:** Easy

Serving size: 4

Ingredients:

- 1 cup of yogurt
- dried fruit mix (almonds, walnuts, hazelnuts, cashews)
- 1 teaspoon of honey
- 1/4 cup of oats
- 1 yellow apple, cut into 8 wedges
- 1 ounce of blackberries

Directions:

Finely chop the dried fruit with a food processor. In a large bowl, put the yogurt and combine the dried fruit with the oats. Add the apple and blackberries. Mix with honey and serve cool.

Nutritional Values: Calories: 70 kcal / Carbohydrates 10g / Protein 12g / Fat 1g / Sugar 3g

Fancy Spelt Bread

Total time: 70 mins / **Prep Time** 20 mins / **Cooking time:** 50 mins / **Difficulty:** Easy

Serving size: 8

Ingredients:

- 4 cups of flour
- salt
- 1/2 cup of shredded walnuts
- brewer's yeast
- 3 tablespoons of red sour cherry jam

Directions:

In a large bowl, prepare the dough by mixing the flour with the salt and yeast. Then, gently start pouring the water. Usually, the necessary quantity corresponds to half of the flour. Knead with your hands or a mixer until you get the desired consistency. When the dough starts to take shape, add the chopped walnuts. Keep the dough and let it rise in a not-too-hot and dry place for about 1 hour. When ready, give one or two large shapes and bake in a preheated oven at 400 ° F for about 45-50 minutes. In the end, wait for the bread to cool, cut it in half, and spread the black cherry jam inside. Serve.

Nutritional Values: Calories: 92 kcal / Carbohydrates 34g / Protein 18g / Fat 0g / Sugar 2g

Lemon Ice Cream

Total time: 8 hours / **Prep Time** 6 hours / **Cooking time:** 10 mins / **Difficulty:** Easy

Serving size: 4

Ingredients:

- 1 cup of heavy cream
- 2 cups of sugar
- 2 cups of carob flour
- juice of 3 lemons

Directions:

In a small saucepan, melt the cream with the sugar and the carob flour. The mixture should not boil but rather be hot. Let it rest for about 6 hours, and then add the lemon juice. Mix without forming lumps. Put the mixture in a friendly freezer in a bowl and stir every 30 minutes. Enjoy it after at least 4 hours of cold.

Nutritional Values: Calories: 115 kcal / Carbohydrates 40g / Protein 20g / Fat 4g / Sugar 12g

Almond Parfait

Total time: 8 hours / **Prep Time** 10 / **Cooking time:** 10 mins / **Difficulty:** Easy

Serving size: 4

Ingredients:

- 1/2 cup of chopped almonds
- ½ cup of sugar
- 3 ounces of cream for desserts
- 1/2 cup of almond milk
- 1/2 cup peeled dry biscuits

Directions:

In a pan, toast the almonds briefly for about 10 minutes. When finished, set aside. Put the cream in a glass dish and mix it with the almond milk and sugar. Add the cookies and shredded almonds. Store in the freezer overnight. Serve

Nutritional Values: Calories: 145 kcal / Carbohydrates 36g / Protein 25g / Fat 19g / Sugar 18g

Nut Cream

Total time: 25 mins / **Prep Time** 15 / **Cooking time:** 10 mins / **Difficulty:** Easy

Serving size: 10

Ingredients:

- 1/2 cup of shelled hazelnuts
- 1 ounce of sugar
- 1 teaspoon of unsweetened cocoa
- 2 tablespoons of seed oil
- 1 cup of dark chocolate

Directions:

Toast the hazelnuts in a saucepan for a few minutes,

stirring briefly. Put them in a blender and blend. Make sure to grind all the hazelnuts. As soon as the hazelnuts release liquid, add the sugar and blend again. Now put everything in a bowl and add the cocoa. Mix gently. Finally, melt the chocolate in a saucepan in a bain-marie. Mix it with a spatula to the previous mixture as soon as it becomes liquid. Put your cream in a glass jar and close with a lid. Store in the refrigerator.

Nutritional Values: Calories: 175 kcal / Carbohydrates 20g / Protein 10g / Fat 40g / Sugar 30g

Avocado Chips

Total time: 35 mins / **Prep Time** 15 mins / **Cooking time:** 20 mins / **Difficulty:** Easy

Serving size: 15

Ingredients:

- 3 ripe avocados, peeled and seedless

- 2 eggs

- 1/2 cup of breadcrumbs

- a pinch of salt

- Fry oil

Directions:

In a dish, put the crumb with the salt, and in a bowl, break the eggs. Cut the avocado into small slices and try not to make them too thick so that they cook sooner. Now dip each piece first in the liquid egg, then in the salty crumb, and set aside. Put the oil in a saucepan and heat. When it is hot, completely dip every slice of breaded avocado and cook it for about 15-20 minutes. When finished, place them in a bowl with paper towels. Serve.

Alternatively, you can use the air fryer by placing the breaded avocado slices directly into the basket and cooking at 390 ° F for 10 minutes per side.

Nutritional Values: Calories: 120 kcal / Carbohydrates 14g / Protein 18g / Fat 22g / Fiber 38g

Conversion Chart

COOKING CONVERSION CHART

Measurement

CUP	ONCES	MILLILITERS	TABLESPOONS
8 cup	64 oz	1895 ml	128
6 cup	48 oz	1420 ml	96
5 cup	40 oz	1180 ml	80
4 cup	32 oz	960 ml	64
2 cup	16 oz	480 ml	32
1 cup	8 oz	240 ml	16
3/4 cup	6 oz	177 ml	12
2/3 cup	5 oz	158 ml	11
1/2 cup	4 oz	118 ml	8
3/8 cup	3 oz	90 ml	6
1/3 cup	2.5 oz	79 ml	5.5
1/4 cup	2 oz	59 ml	4
1/8 cup	1 oz	30 ml	3
1/16 cup	1/2 oz	15 ml	1

Temperature

FAHRENHEIT	CELSIUS
100 °F	37 °C
150 °F	65 °C
200 °F	93 °C
250 °F	121 °C
300 °F	150 °C
325 °F	160 °C
350 °F	180 °C
375 °F	190 °C
400 °F	200 °C
425 °F	220 °C
450 °F	230 °C
500 °F	260 °C
525 °F	274 °C
550 °F	288 °C

Weight

IMPERIAL	METRIC
1/2 oz	15 g
1 oz	29 g
2 oz	57 g
3 oz	85 g
4 oz	113 g
5 oz	141 g
6 oz	170 g
8 oz	227 g
10 oz	283 g
12 oz	340 g
13 oz	369 g
14 oz	397 g
15 oz	425 g
1 lb	453 g

30 Day Meal Plan

Days	Breakfast	Lunch	Dinner	Dessert/snack
1	Mushroom Quinoa	Roasted Tofu with coconut Milk	Cilantro lime quinoa	Chocolate Cookies
2	Banana Chips	Sweet and Sour Potatoes with Meat	Spinach Quinoa	Detox Dried Fruit with Chestnut Honey
3	Coconut cream pancakes	Stuffed Peppers	Pineapple and Carrot Salad	Coconut Cream Bars
4	Mayo Salad	Baked Fish	Peppers Pizza	Almond Cake
5	Bread with alkaline vegetable cream	Onion Omelette	Healthy Broccoli and Asparagus	Chia Breadstick and cracker
6	Vegetables Quinoa	Chickpeas and vegetables	Baked Pumpkin	Kiwi with Dried Fruit
7	Zucchini Muffin	Boiled Chicken	Pumpkin Risotto	Homemade Protein Bars
8	carrot juice	Veal with mango sauce	Mixed Legumes Soup	Orange and Pumpkin Salad
9	Potato Salad	Baked Tomatoes	Zucchini Risotto	Banana and nuts Muffin
10	Banana Porridge	Vegetable Hash	Pineapple and Coconut	Strawberry Salad
11	Breakfast salad	Champignon Omelette	Chicken Muffin	STRAWBERRY JAM
12	Butternut Squash	Chicken with Sweet Potatoes	Raw Rainbow Vegetables	Biscuits bars
13	Alkaline Minestrone	Mix Grilled Vegetables	Fresh fruit and Vanilla	Simple Anti-inflammatory Biscuit
14	Lemon Smoothie	Vegetables and Lentils	Vegetables with green toppings	Chickpea Humus
15	Cabbage Salad	Artichokes and	Champignon	Cereal with

		quinoa	Risotto	Yogurt
16	Red Thai Vegetable curry	Stuffed Eggplant	Roasted Zucchini	Coconut Chips
17	Zucchini Home Fries	Baked Onions and Potatoes	Sweet Pepper Cream	Pear and Apple Extract
18	Green Smoothie	Spicy Meat	Tomato Cream with Quinoa	Apple Cake
19	Hemp Seed Porridge	Mix Fermented Vegetables	Green Sweet Creamy Zucchini	Fermented Zucchini
20	Mayo Salad	Asparagus Omelette	Scrambled tofu e tomato	Coconut and Almond Biscuits
21	Potato Salad	Roasted Eggplant	Grilled Tofu	Purifying Juice
22	Lemon Smoothie	Mashed cauliflower	Breaded Chicken	Apple Muffin
23	Cabbage Salad	Quinoa and Oatmeal	Spicy Chicken	Apple Alkaline Cream
24	Zucchini Home Fries	Breaded Chicken	baked Sea Bass	Avocado Salad
25	Breakfast salad	Italian Chicken	Boiled Octopus	Yogurt and dried Fruit
26	Zucchini Muffin	Pasta with Seafood	Potatoes Salad	Fancy Spelt Bread
27	Green Smoothie	Roasted Salmon	Healthy Anti-inflammatory Salad	Lemon Ice Cream
28	Potato Salad	Pork with Green Sauce	Fresh Spelled Avocado Salad	Almond Parfait
29	Cabbage Salad	Meat with peppers	Roasted Pepper Cream	Nut Cream
30	Zucchini Home Fries	Rocket Fish	Tomato Cream with Quinoa	Avocado Chips

CONCLUSION:

Congratulations! You have completed our journey through the anti-inflammatory diet, exploring the basic principles, foods, and nutrients with anti-inflammatory power and the importance of lifestyle to support your overall health and well-being.

The anti-inflammatory diet is more than just a food choice; it is a holistic health approach involving the body and mind. Throughout this journey, you have learned how some foods can contribute to chronic inflammation while others can help us fight it. You have discovered antioxidants, omega-3 fatty acids, and spices that can significantly reduce inflammation in your body.

But we don't stop there. This book contains a treasure trove of tasty and nutritious recipes to make your anti-inflammatory diet healthy and delicious. We have included a 30-day eating plan to guide you through an excellent start on your journey to an anti-inflammatory diet. Each day, you will experience a variety of dishes, ingredients, and flavors, all while working toward your health and inflammation control.

However, remember that the journey to wellness is an individual one. Each of you will have different needs and goals; the key to success is listening to your body. Take the time to observe how your inflammation levels may change over time by monitoring your health, weight, energy, and vitality. Adjust your diet and lifestyle to suit your needs, and feel free to experiment with the foods and recipes you like best.

Remember to keep exploring and educating yourself about food and lifestyle choices that help you achieve your health goals. Maintain a balanced and sustainable approach to maintain the benefits of the anti-inflammatory diet over time.

Finally, if you have questions or need additional support, remember that I, Rachel Rodriguez, and other health professionals are here to help you. Consulting with a nutritionist or health professional can provide additional personalized guidance and answers to your questions.

I wish you the best on this journey to a healthier life with less inflammation. Be compassionate with yourself, celebrate your successes, and continue to invest in your health. May this anti-inflammatory diet lead you to a bright future of well-being, vitality, and joy. Enjoy your journey!

Made in the USA
Middletown, DE
21 August 2023